you are what you eat ™

Total Health Overhaul

by
Carina Norris

First published in Great Britain in 2008 by
Virgin Books Ltd
Thames Wharf Studios
Rainville Road
London
W6 9HA

A catalogue record for this book is available from the British Library.

ISBN 978 0 7535 1375 0

The paper used in this book is a natural, recyclable product made from wood grown in sustainable forests. The manufacturing process conforms to the regulations of the country of origin.

Designed by Virgin Books Ltd

Printed and bound by Firmengruppe APPL, aprinta druck, Germany

All photography copyright © Shutterstock, except p215 copyright © Corbis

you are what you eat ™

Contents

INTRODUCTION

Get ready for a new you.

You care about your health, and realise that the food you eat is more than just 'fuel' – you've shown you appreciate that simply by picking up this book. Food has a huge bearing on how you feel right now, and also your long-term health. Get it right, and you can enjoy plenty of energy and reduce your risk of illnesses, from coughs and sniffles to serious conditions like heart disease and cancer. Get it wrong, and you'll feel rough, and your body will feel old before its time.

New beginnings can be daunting, and perhaps you're not quite sure where to start – particularly if you think your diet is pretty dreadful at the moment. You might believe the task is just too huge, or that you can't face a lifetime without your favourite foods.

But healthy eating needn't be scary – it can be practical and fun. You don't need to be an expert cook, or spend hours in the kitchen – you've got better things to do with your time! You don't need to spend a fortune on exotic or expensive ingredients. In fact, you'll be able to buy most of the ingredients in this book from the supermarket. And you don't have to exist on rabbit food, and dull, tasteless meals. Life is for living, and food is for enjoying!

This book is all about making things easy for you. And in case you're wavering about whether giving up your old, bad habits is worthwhile, we'll be explaining just what's in it for you.

Knowing just why the You Are What You Eat way works so well will help, too. Once you understand exactly what those greasy chips are going to do to your arteries and your waistline, it will be so much easier to say no!

And because it's not fair to deprive you of your old favourites without giving you something just as tasty in their place, this book is packed with tempting recipes and meal ideas to fit in with your new way of eating. For example, from now on you won't have greasy fried chips – you'll have home-made chunky oven chips, baked in their skins, instead. Just as tasty – and much, much healthier!

Now that you've decided you want to change (and congratulations, by the way) you'll want to get started. And you'll want to see results quickly – you're only human, after all. In the past, you might have been tempted to go on a crash diet, cutting out everything that's 'naughty', and existing on little more than willpower and fresh air.

Slow down! Crash diets aren't healthy, and you will set yourself up to fail. You'll be hungry, you'll feel miserable and deprived, you'll soon become deficient in vital nutrients, and your health will suffer. You'll feel discouraged and, likely as not, you'll lapse, and feel guilty as well.

Healthy eating, on the other hand, isn't a quick fix – but it is a lasting solution.

This book is all about a new start that will lead to healthier habits to last for the rest of your life. We will lead you through an eight-week plan to set you on the nutritional straight and narrow. It's a step-by-step guide to a healthy diet, full of tasty real food. You won't find any of the fatty, sugary props you may have relied on before – they're replaced with healthier substitutes. It may seem quite strict at first – particularly if you were used to eating badly – but it's by no means a crash diet. For a start, it's not specifically a weight-loss diet – though if you were eating too much of the wrong foods before, you'll find you do lose weight.

Many strict diets, especially those aiming for rapid weight loss, involve a drastic cutting in calories, and sometimes the removal of entire food groups. This kind of dietary manipulation can be dangerous, because less food and less variety means less nutrients. Rest assured, the eating plan in this book contains all the nutrients you need to keep you in tiptop health.

And you'll be eating plenty of food. In fact, you may feel that you're eating more than before. While junk food is generally high in fat and calories, the foods we recommend are low in them – but high in taste. And the foods in your new eating plan are low in salt and sugar, but high in vitamins and minerals, so you can enjoy them with a clear conscience.

The first four weeks in our plan are a kick-start – four weeks is long enough for you to really start feeling the benefits of your new way of life. Within days you'll have more energy. By a couple of weeks, you could find yourself feeling more easy-going and less moody. And in a month, you might even have shed a few pounds and find your belt needs to be nipped in a notch or two.

Seeing real progress is just what you need to keep you motivated. When life feels this good, who needs junk food for comfort? But what if you feel that life just wouldn't be worth living if you could never enjoy a cup of coffee, or a slice of cake, ever again?

Don't worry – they're not going to be banned! Once you've seen what just four weeks of healthy eating can do for you, we're confident that you won't want to go back to 'bad old ways'. But there's no reason why you shouldn't be free to enjoy the occasional slap-up meal out with friends. When someone offers around a box of chocolates, you don't always have to say no. And there's no harm in the occasional cappuccino and biscotti while you're out shopping. You just have to realise that this kind of eating isn't a way of life any more.

Provided you eat healthily most of the time, it's OK to relax once in a while. And for that reason, we'll explain how you can do this, with helpful hints, and a four-week 'Forever Plan' to carry on with.

So, prepare to dive into a new way of eating – and get ready to feel the benefits of a New You.

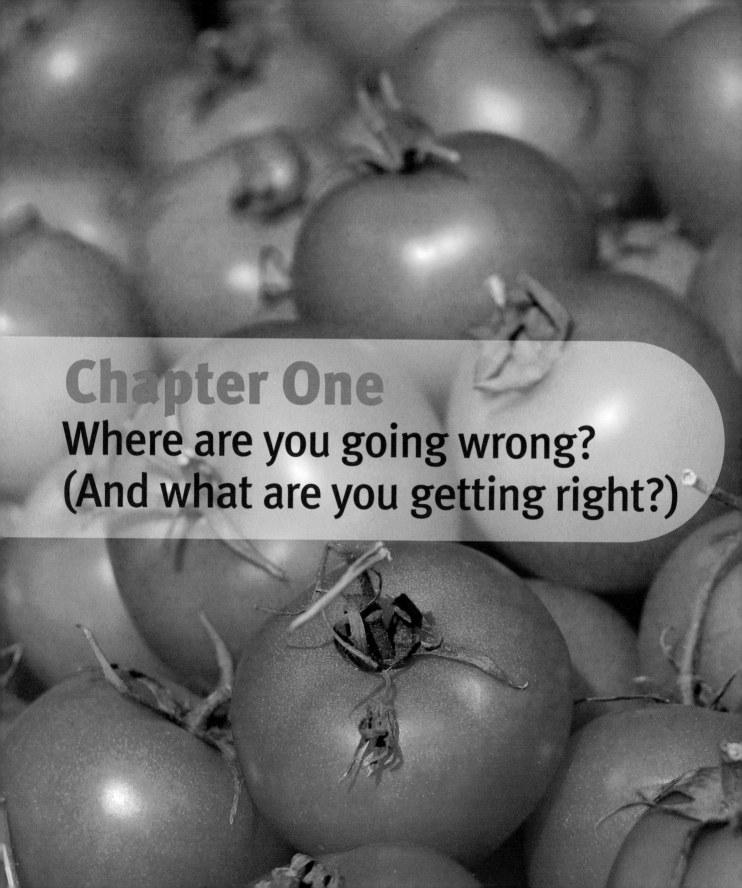

Chapter One
Where are you going wrong? (And what are you getting right?)

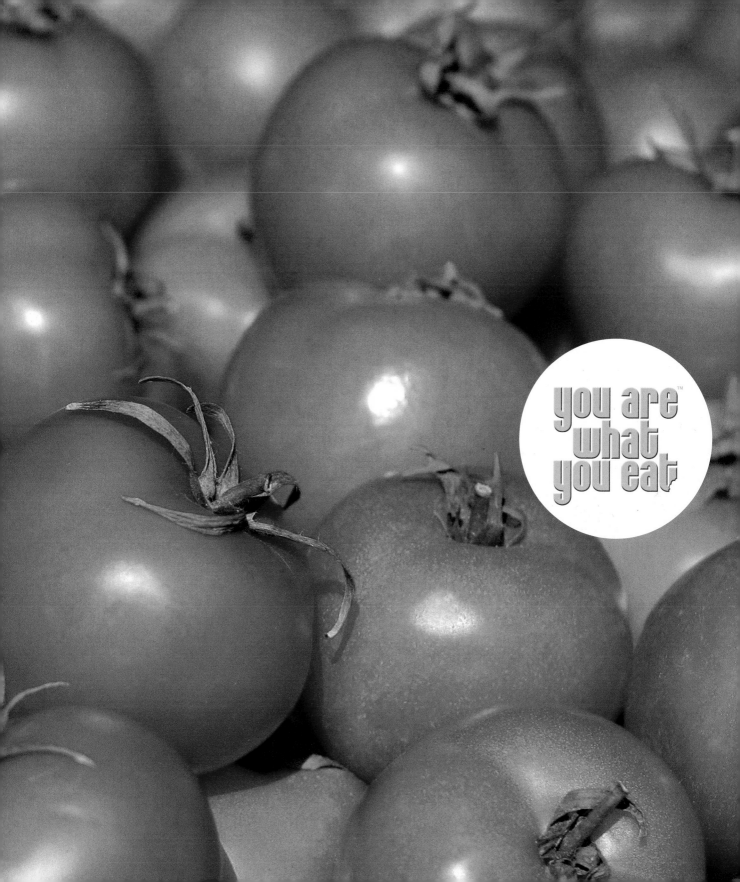

you are what you eat™

Getting Started

Basically, our diets (and lifestyles) go wrong when they get out of balance:

- We eat (and do) the things we shouldn't
- We don't eat (or do) the things we should

Put like that, it's simple! And this book will explain just what you should and shouldn't be eating, and why. To make things simple, we've got helpful tips to painlessly cut down the unhealthy things in our diet, and eat more of the healthy foods – practical advice that will fit into your busy lifestyle.

We'll also help you to sort out your exercise and drinking habits.

In order to feel and look your best, you need to be eating healthily, and getting enough exercise – it's not enough to just do one or the other.

Perhaps you're already quite active, but your junk-food habits are holding you back, sapping your energy and preventing you from achieving your full fitness potential. Or maybe you eat fairly healthily, but you never manage to fit in time for any exercise, so you might find running up a flight of stairs or dashing for a bus leaves you out of breath.

Even if you feel you're already doing all right in the eating and exercise departments, there's probably still room for improvement – none of us are perfect! Follow the advice in this book to move up from feeling just 'OK' to being full of life and bouncing with health.

What if you've let your diet **and** your exercise habits slip? It's nothing to be ashamed of. You just need to decide to change, arm yourself with the knowledge to get yourself motivated (and stay motivated) – then get started!

Assess Your Starting Point

Before you get started you need to know your starting point – otherwise you won't be able to judge your progress.

Watching the progress you're making – and feeling the benefits – is the best motivator in the world!

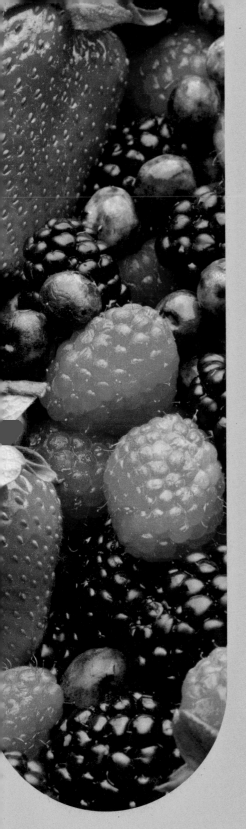

First, let's take a close look at where your own personal nutritional pitfalls lie. Perhaps you have a particularly sweet tooth, or a craving for crisps. Or maybe you like 'chips with everything'. Perhaps your social life revolves around evenings at the pub with friends, followed by a takeaway meal.

Your food diary

Your best ally in sorting out your nutritional bad habits is a 'food diary' – it enables you to pinpoint exactly where your weaknesses are. Writing down what you eat can be a real eye-opener. Scientific research has shown that when people ask us what we've eaten over the course of the last week, or even just the previous day, our estimates are far less accurate than if we'd written the foods down at the time we ate them.

And interestingly, it's not just a case of poor memories across the board. People are far more likely to forget about less healthy foods – the ones that are high in fat and sugar – than the healthy ones we know we should be eating. And it's all too easy to forget snacks! We're not being dishonest when we do this – it's natural and unconscious, and it's been scientifically proven to occur.

So, what you need for a more accurate record of what you eat is to find yourself a notebook (choose a small, neat one that you'll like writing in, because you're going to be carrying it around with you for a while!) and divide each page into three columns. (We've provided an example of a food diary on page 218 to show you the idea, along with some helpful tips on how we'd interpret it.)

At the beginning of each day, write the date and day of the week. Then you need to write down everything you eat or drink. In the first column write the time that you eat it, in the second write what it was that you ate, and the third column is for any relevant notes. For example, you might note down why you ate something – perhaps you were really hungry, bored, waiting for someone, or maybe it was through habit – you always have a couple of biscuits at eleven o'clock. You could also make a note of how the food made you feel – a cup of coffee might make you jittery, or a big meal could make you feel tired afterwards.

It might sound like an awful lot of effort, but give it a try – it really is worth it. As well as giving you a real insight into the way you eat at the moment, it can also help you plan for the future.

Using your food diary

Once you've filled in your food diary for a week or so, you can work out where your weaknesses lie, so you'll be better able to put them right.

Spot the 'danger foods'

First, scan the pages for unhealthy foods – things like:

- Crisps
- Chips
- Other fried foods
- Sweets
- Chocolate
- Fizzy drinks
- Alcohol
- Fast food
- Ice cream
- Cakes and pastries
- Pies and pasties
- Biscuits

Some of these foods are allowable in small quantities as a treat – but if you see them cropping up again and again, you know they're a 'danger food' for you, and you need to cut down drastically.

Check your meal patterns

Then look at when you're eating. Do you manage to give yourself regular meal times, without waiting too long before eating? Or are you grabbing meals, eating on the run, or even skipping meals? If you eat regularly, you're less likely to reach for an unhealthy snack to tide you over between meals. But if your mealtimes are haphazard, your blood-sugar and energy levels will get out of kilter, and you're far more likely to succumb to the temptation of a chocolate biscuit or packet of crisps when your energy levels fall or you're feeling peckish.

Snacking habits

Also, look at your snacking habits. There's nothing wrong with snacking – snacks are a good way of maintaining steady energy levels and resisting the unhealthy temptations we've just mentioned. You just need to ensure that you eat the right kind of snacks.

Bad snacks provide short-lived energy, and contribute little to good nutrition. Examples of bad snacks are:

- Chocolate bars
- Sweets
- Ice cream
- Cakes and pastries
- Biscuits
- Crisps

Good snacks, on the other hand, maintain your energy levels, while also providing essential nutrients. Examples of good snacks are:

- A piece of fruit, such as an apple, orange, pear, banana, small bunch of grapes
- A couple of oatcakes
- A small tub of low-fat cottage cheese with pineapple
- A tablespoon of raisins with a few unsalted nuts
- A wholemeal currant bun

What about your drinking?

What do you drink, how much, and when? You should have at least eight glasses of water (approximately 1.5 litres) per day. What else do you drink? Milk? Tea and coffee? Fizzy drinks? Alcohol? You need to ensure that you get enough fluids, yet avoid too much alcohol, caffeine or sugar in your drinks. You'll learn more about the best (and worst) things to drink later in this book.

Look for the 'good foods'

In Chapter 2 you'll find the foods you really should be eating more of – look through your food diary to check your intake of healthy foods like fruit and vegetables, nuts and seeds, lean meat, fish, low-fat dairy products, wholegrains and healthy unsaturated fats.

Why do you eat?

Take a look at your notes about why you eat, and how it made you feel. Do you often eat foods you shouldn't when you're bored, lonely or unhappy? If so, these problems will make sticking to a healthy diet more difficult. If you can get to the root of these other troubles and solve them, you won't have to turn to food as a crutch to keep you going or make you feel better.

But don't think that having a less than perfect life gives you an excuse not to at least try to eat healthily. Eating a nutritious diet can give you more energy and make you feel and look better, which will give you an extra boost in sorting out the rest of your life.

Also, look for any danger triggers that make you more likely to reach for a less than healthy 'foody prop'. Perhaps you're a woman who craves sweet things at certain times of the month? Or maybe your diet goes to pieces when the children have exams at school? Or do you rely on junk food when you're busy and under pressure at work? If you know the danger points, you'll be forewarned, and better able to avoid falling off the healthy-eating wagon.

Filling in a food diary for a week or two casts a spotlight on your eating habits. Some people find it's helpful to continue to keep a food diary for longer than this – it helps them to keep track of what they're eating, and makes them feel 'accountable'. You're less likely to eat a chocolate muffin if you know you've got to write it down in your diary! Keeping a long-term diary also enables you to look back and see your progress – a great motivator!

Even if you don't want to fill in a diary all the time, it's well worth writing down a few days every couple of months – just to see how well you're doing (or whether you've let your good intentions slip!).

Fitness Matters!

Eating a healthy diet is only part of the story – you also need exercise to keep your body strong and healthy.

Our bodies are designed to be active – we're not made to be couch potatoes, and that's where a lot of our health problems begin. When you start exercising, it may feel like hard work at first, but it will get easier as your fitness improves. Don't feel discouraged if you're an exercise novice – it's when you're just starting out that the improvements in your health are most dramatic. Someone who's never exercised before, then decides to take a gentle walk each day, will see far more noticeable benefits than someone who already goes to the gym five times a week and adds a new exercise to their routine.

And fitness is a holistic concept – you need a variety of different kinds in order to get the maximum benefits. In that way, it's like healthy eating! It also works alongside healthy eating, to give you the best all-round health, and that all-important feel-good factor.

Just as you need a balanced diet, you need 'balanced exercise'. If you concentrate on one kind of exercise to the exclusion of all others, you won't gain the all-round fitness that brings so many health benefits and makes you feel great. For example, what's the point of a man having terrific muscles, if he can't run for a bus? And even if a woman is fit enough to run a marathon, it's not much practical use if her muscle strength isn't enough to easily lift her toddler into the car. And although strength and stamina are all very important, being so inflexible that you can't do things like bend down to tie your shoelaces makes life a lot more difficult. Flexibility also helps to make other forms of exercise easier, and reduces your risk of injuries.

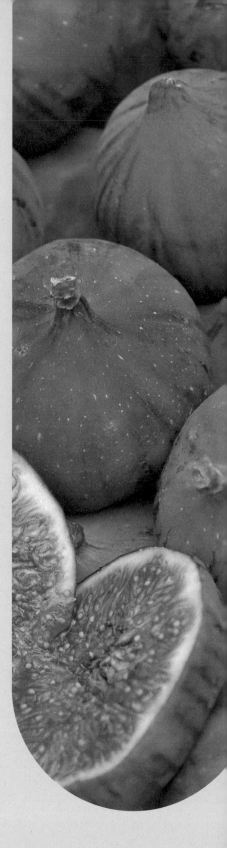

You need a combination of all three types of exercise, and this book will show you how to incorporate them into your life.

You can divide exercise into three types:

- **Cardiovascular exercise** – to keep your heart and lungs strong and healthy. It helps with everyday activities like running up stairs.
- **Strength exercise** – to build and maintain your muscles and bones. This helps with everyday activities like lifting heavy shopping and mowing the lawn.
- **Flexibility exercise** – for ease of movement throughout life. This helps with everyday activities like reaching up to high shelves and dealing with zips and buttons behind your back.

The whole picture

Addressing your diet and exercise habits can have a huge bearing on your health and wellbeing – but they're not the whole story. There are other areas of your lifestyle where you could be holding yourself back, or even putting your life at risk.

Smoking: If you smoke, quitting is almost certainly the most important thing you could do for your health – and also the health of those around you. You'll reduce your risk of heart disease, stroke, cancer and lung disease, and feel much better, too. But it's not easy, so get help. For more information: www.gosmokefree.co.uk

Stress: Too much stress suppresses the immune system, raises your blood pressure, and slows the healing process when you're injured. If you can't remove the cause of the stress, you need to find coping and relaxing mechanisms. A friendly ear can help, as can exercise, either vigorous, or more relaxing forms like yoga.

Sleep: Not getting enough sleep can seriously affect your quality of life, leaving you tired, fuzzy-headed, and more likely to have an accident. Research has even linked lack of sleep with an increased risk of obesity. For more information on getting a good night's sleep, visit: www.sleepcouncil.com

Tests: Take advantage of any tests your GP offers, such as blood pressure, cholesterol, and blood glucose (for diabetes), as well as any 'well woman' or 'well man' tests or clinics available. Problems caught early can be nipped in the bud, and these tests could save your life.

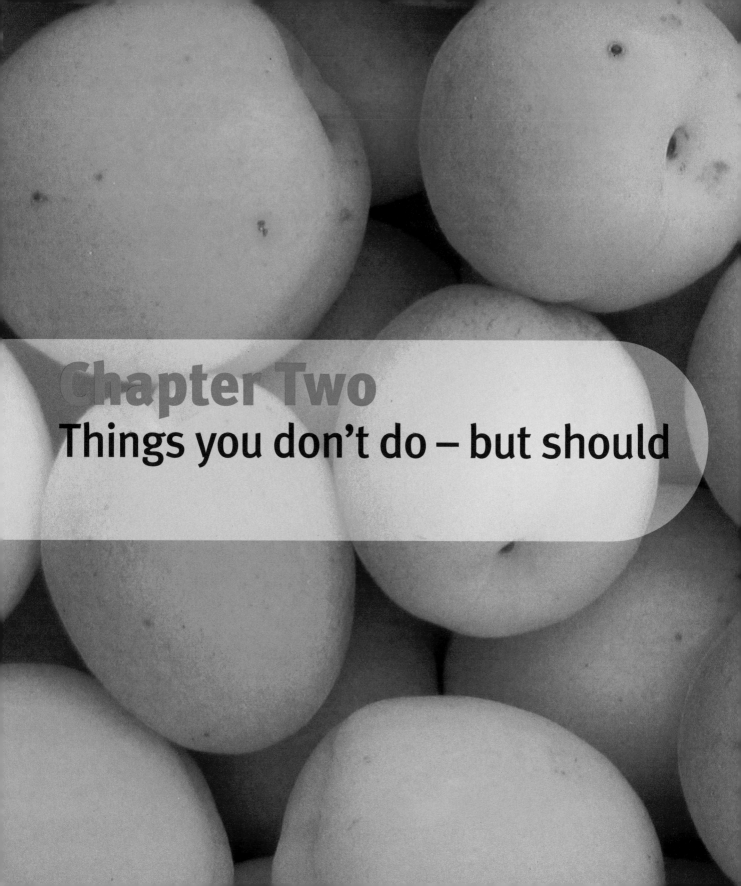

Chapter Two
Things you don't do – but should

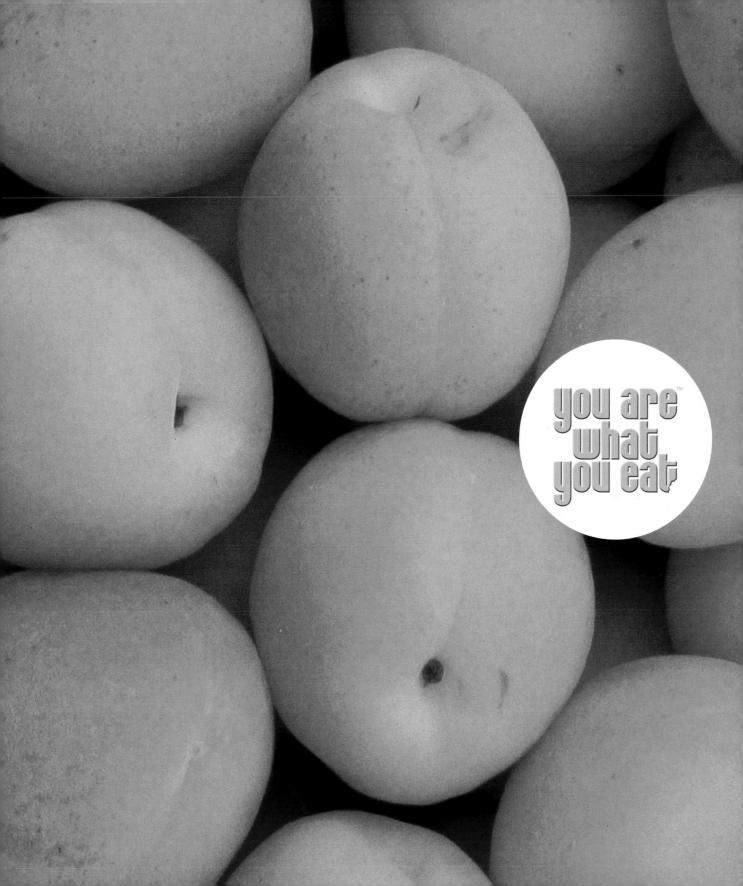

you are what you eat™

Maintain a Healthy Weight

One of the most important things you can do in order to feel great and boost your health is maintain a healthy weight. We're not talking about some super-skinny so-called ideal you may see on the catwalk or the pages of a glossy magazine – that's unrealistic and unhealthy. We mean a healthy weight that's right for you. Unfortunately there's no magic formula. But it is possible, by taking into account a variety of factors, to figure out an estimate of what's best for you.

What's your perfect weight?

The most commonly used way of measuring whether someone is underweight, a healthy weight, overweight or obese (seriously overweight) is the body mass index, or BMI. This is basically how heavy you are for your height.

Here's how to work it out:

1. Measure your height in metres, and square it (i.e. height x height)
2. Measure your weight in kilograms
3. Divide your weight by your height squared

So, take for example a 1.64m (5 foot 4 inches) woman who weighs 65kg (10 stone). To calculate her BMI:

1. Multiply height x height – 1.64 x 1.64 = 2.69
2. Divide weight by (height x height) – 65/2.69 = 24.16

BMI below 18.5   =   underweight
BMI 18.5 to 25   =   healthy weight
BMI 25 to 29   =   overweight
BMI over 30   =   obese

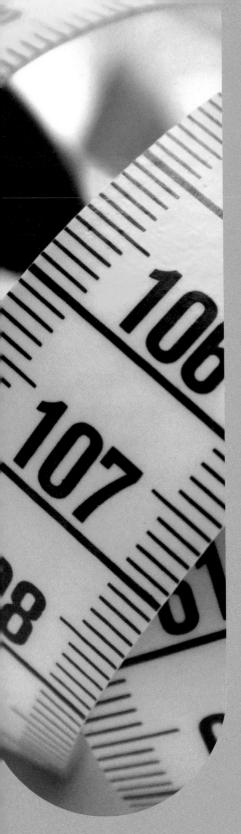

So, the woman in our example calculation, with a BMI of approximately 24, falls within the healthy weight category.

The main problem with BMI is that it isn't accurate for anyone whose ratio of body muscle to fat is far from 'average'. This includes children, pregnant women, the elderly and conditioned athletes.

For example, athletes and sportsmen and women can have extremely low body-fat percentages – they're very high in muscle. Muscle is heavier than fat, and since BMI measures how heavy you are for your height, they seem very heavy indeed. This makes their BMI look unhealthy, when in fact they're extremely fit.

Waist to hip ratio

Perhaps a better way to determine whether you're a healthy weight is to look at your waist to hip ratio, since this is a measure of how much fat you're storing around your middle.

This is important, because your waistline is not a healthy place to store fat. The problem is that it's easier for stored belly fat to get into the bloodstream, contributing to clogged arteries, and hence your risk of heart disease and stroke. It also increases your risk of getting type 2 diabetes.

Although having fat around your bottom and thighs may make you feel less attractive, it's actually less of a health risk than belly fat.

Where you store your fat is largely determined by your genes – you have the tendency to be either an 'apple-shaped' or 'pear-shaped' person:

● Apple shapes: Store fat around their waists, and are more likely to be men. Higher risk of cardiovascular disease and type 2 diabetes.

● Pear shapes: Store fat around their hips and thighs, and are more likely to be women. Lower risk of cardiovascular disease and type 2 diabetes.

Here's how to discover whether your belly could be a health risk:

1. Measure your waist
2. Measure your hips
3. Divide the waist measurement by the hip measurement

These are the danger levels (giving you a significantly higher health risk):

- Ratio of over 0.85 for women
- Ratio of over 0.90 for men

An even easier method of measuring whether you have an unhealthy amount of belly fat is to simply measure your waist. The danger levels are:

- Waist measuring more than 88cm/35 inches for a woman
- Waist measuring more than 100cm/40 inches for a man

Unfortunately, you can't change your genetic tendency to lay down fat on either your waist or your hips and thighs. But if you know you've a tendency to lay down fat in the 'apple shape' location, it makes it all the more important for you to watch your weight, and keep fit and active.

Make it practical

Measure your BMI, and waist to hip ratio. Is it higher than it should be? If so, you'll benefit even more than most from embarking on our eating and exercise plan.

If you're extremely overweight, or over the 'at risk' level for waist to hip ratio, it's a good idea to make an appointment with your doctor or practice nurse. They can take your blood pressure, check your blood cholesterol, and measure your blood-sugar level (to check for diabetes). This way you'll catch any potential problems early on, when you can nip them in the bud. Your medical practice may also be able to put you in touch with a dietician, for nutritional advice that's tailored to your particular health needs.

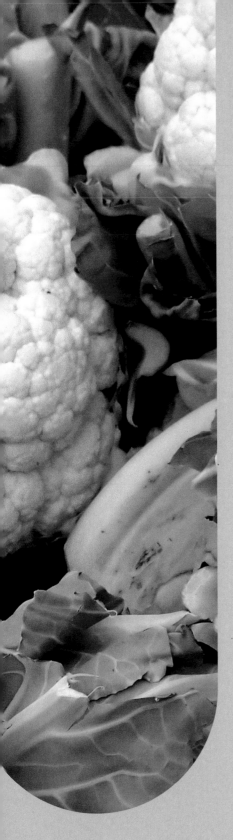

Healthy Eating
Are you getting enough?

You'll probably be pleased to hear that eating the You Are What You Eat way isn't all about telling you what NOT to eat. Although there are certainly foods we should be cutting down or out, it's far better to concentrate on the delicious and nutritious foods we should all be eating more of.

We need to emphasise the positive – it's much easier to revamp your diet for the better if you concentrate on eating more of the good things, than dwelling on all the things you shouldn't eat any more and making yourself miserable. Far too many people who are trying to improve their diets try really hard to cut out the 'bad foods', but forget all about what they should be eating more of.

Studies have also proven that people who make a real effort to eat more of the healthy foods, such as fruit and vegetables, find that their intake of unhealthy foods (such as those high in fat and added sugars) decreases naturally. And that can't be bad!

Unfortunately, however, many of us are remarkably bad at making sure we eat enough of the tasty and nutritious fuel our bodies are crying out for. We ignore the fact that neglecting healthy foods throws our diets out of kilter as well.

How good are you at making sure you eat enough:

- Fruit
- Vegetables
- Nuts and seeds
- Oily fish
- Wholegrain carbohydrates
- Water

Most of us fall short in at least one of them! But it's easy – and no hardship – to get it right, and reap the benefits. And in this section, we'll show you how.

Overweight and undernourished

It's ironic that, when so many of us are overweight, we're also likely to be undernourished. A worrying proportion of the population fall short of their daily requirements for several nutrients, especially minerals.

The most recent National Diet and Nutrition Survey revealed that:

- A significant proportion of the UK population don't get the recommended amount of several vitamins, especially vitamin A, the B vitamins and vitamin C.
- Young adults (under 34), especially women, are most likely to fall short of their vitamin and mineral intakes. The most 'problematic' nutrients proved to be vitamin A, vitamin B2, iron, potassium and magnesium.
- Over 90 per cent of women under the age of 50 have iron intakes below the recommended daily amount. Nearly half of women under 50 have iron intakes below the 'bare minimum' level that's only enough for a tiny proportion of the population – those who naturally have very low needs. All this means that a large proportion of women are at risk from iron deficiency anaemia, with its unpleasant symptoms of weakness, tiredness and lethargy.
- The average young woman's intake of calcium is below the recommended amount. Calcium is particularly important for young women, since the years before your thirties are the time when most bone mass is built up, reducing the risk of osteoporosis later in life.
- A significant number of women don't get enough folic acid. This is a problem for pregnant women and those planning a baby, because this vitamin reduces the risk of neural-tube defects such as spina bifida in their babies. Not getting enough folic acid may also be linked with an increased risk of heart disease.
- Nearly half of the adult UK population has an inadequate intake of zinc, which is needed to support the immune system, and for a healthy reproductive system.
- Nearly three-quarters of women have magnesium intakes below the recommended level. Around a quarter of women aged 19 to 34 have magnesium intakes below the 'bare minimum' cut-off point that's only sufficient for a very few people (those with low requirements). Magnesium is required for a huge range of chemical reactions in the body.

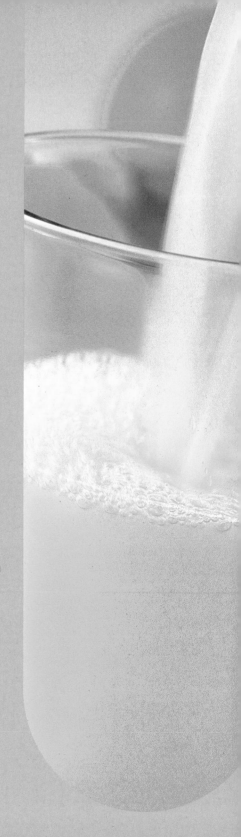

Thankfully, it's easy to ensure that you're not one of these unhealthy statistics. The most common reason for most people failing to hit their nutrient targets is the fact that they don't eat a varied, balanced diet, and in particular they don't eat enough fruit and vegetables – and that's so easy to fix!

How good is your diet?
Answer the questions, and add up the scores in the boxes.

1. How many portions of fruit do you eat each day? (Turn to page 28 if you're not sure how big a portion is.)
a) None   **0**
b) 1   **1**
c) 2   **2**
d) 3 or more   **3**

2. How many portions of vegetables do you eat each day? (Turn to page 28 if you're not sure how big a portion is.)
a) None   **0**
b) 1   **1**
c) 2   **2**
d) 3 or more   **3**

3. How often do you eat fish (any kind, except fried, breaded or battered)?
a) Never   **0**
b) Once every few weeks   **1**
c) 1 or 2 times a week   **2**
d) 3 times or more a week   **3**

4. How often do you eat oily fish (salmon, trout, mackerel, pilchards, sardines or fresh (not tinned) tuna)?
a) Never   **0**
b) Once every few weeks   **1**
c) Once a week   **2**
d) Twice or more a week   **3**

5. How much water do you drink each day?
a) Up to 4 medium glasses   `1`
b) 4 to 8 glasses   `2`
c) 8 or more glasses   `3`

6. What kind of bread do you eat?
a) Don't eat bread   `0`
b) Always white   `0`
c) Usually white, sometimes wholemeal   `1`
d) Usually wholemeal, sometimes white   `2`
e) Always wholemeal   `3`

7. How often do you eat wholegrains (apart from wholemeal bread) – including brown rice, brown pasta, buckwheat, bulghur wheat, porridge oats or oatmeal?
a) Never   `0`
b) Occasionally – twice a week or less   `1`
c) 3 to 6 times a week   `2`
d) Every day   `3`

8. How often do you eat calcium-rich foods, such as milk, yogurt, low-fat cheese, or non-dairy calcium sources such as tofu, tinned fish (where you eat the bones), sesame seeds or dried fruit?
a) Hardly ever   `0`
b) Sometimes, but less than once a day   `1`
c) 1 to 2 times a day   `2`
d) 3 or more times a day   `3`

9. How often do you eat nuts and seeds?
a) Never   `0`
b) Occasionally – twice a week or less   `1`
c) 3 to 6 times a week   `2`
d) Every day   `3`

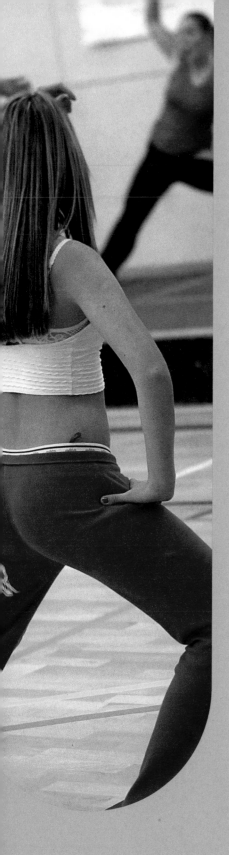

10. How often do you exercise enough to get out of breath, for at least 20 minutes?
a) Never `0`
b) Occasionally – once a week or less `1`
c) 2 to 3 times a week `2`
d) 4 or more times a week `3`

11. How often do you do 'strength exercises', such as weight training at the gym, or using hand- and ankle-weights or doing press-ups and sit-ups at home?
a) Never `0`
b) Occasionally – once a week or less `1`
c) Twice a week `2`
d) Three or more times a week `3`

12. How often do you do stretching exercises, including yoga and Pilates?
a) Never `0`
b) Occasionally – less than once a week `1`
c) Once a week `2`
d) Twice a week or more `3`

Scoring
Add up your scores and see how you did:

0–12: It looks as though you've let your diet or activity levels, and probably both, slip. Don't be discouraged, though, because the only way is up, and if you follow the advice in this book, you'll soon be feeling the benefits.

13–25: There are quite a few areas in your lifestyle that need attention. Perhaps you don't get enough fruit and vegetables, or you've slouched your way into a couch-potato lifestyle. Pay particular attention to the questions you received low scores for, and you'll be rewarded by improved health and energy levels.

25–36: You're doing well! But everyone has an area of weakness or two. Maybe you don't drink enough water, or have never seen the point in strength exercises. Find the questions that stopped you from scoring full marks, and pay particular attention to these areas as you read this book.

Eating enough fruit and vegetables

If you want to eat more healthily, getting more fruit and vegetables inside you is arguably the best thing you can do.

Eating more fruit and veg can:

- Increase your intake of vitamins, especially vitamin C, beta-carotene (a plant chemical which the body converts to vitamin A) and folic acid (one of the B vitamins, important for heart health and vital for pregnant women and those planning a baby).
- Boost your intake of certain minerals, especially potassium (important for maintaining healthy blood pressure).
- Increase your levels of antioxidants, which protect our bodies' cells from damage.
- Supply phytochemicals (plant chemicals) with powerful health benefits, such as reducing your risk of serious chronic diseases such as cancer and heart disease.
- Boost your fibre intake, smoothing the process of digestion, and also reducing your risk of clogged arteries.
- Help you to maintain your weight. The fibre and water in fruit and vegetables fill you up, so you'll be less tempted to eat unhealthy, high-calorie foods.

Different fruit and vegetables contain different vitamins, minerals and phyto-chemicals, and the more varied your fruit and vegetable intake, the more likely you are to get enough of all the different nutrients.

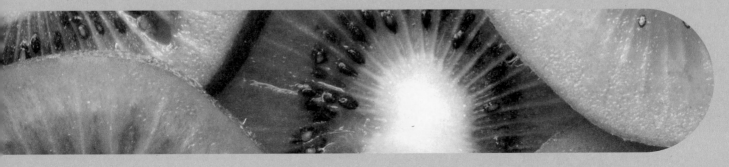

Phytochemicals – your natural health protectors

Plants contain natural health-boosting chemicals, called phytochemicals, which literally means 'plant chemicals'. The vitamins that come from plants are phytochemicals, as are the pigments that give fruit and vegetables their vibrant colours. Many of these pigments act as antioxidants, neutralising harmful molecules called 'free radicals' which damage our bodies' cells.

Phytochemicals have the exciting potential to reduce our risk of illnesses, from the common cold to cancer.

Eat plenty of carrots, broccoli, onions, garlic and tomatoes – these are particularly rich in health-promoting phytochemicals.

There are far too many phytochemicals to list, but here are just a few of the star players:

Allicin – found in onions and garlic.

Anthocyanins – in purple, blue and black fruits, such as beetroot and blueberries.

Beta-carotene – this pigment makes carrots orange, but it's also found in other orange fruit and vegetables such as sweet potatoes, apricots and cantaloupe melons.

Bioflavonoids – from citrus fruits such as oranges, lemons and grapefruits.

Glucosinolates – these are found in vegetables such as cabbage and broccoli.

Lutein – you can find it in kale, spinach, broccoli, and also kiwi fruits!

Lycopene – found mainly in tomatoes, but also in some other red fruits such as pink grapefruit and watermelon.

Organo-sulphur compounds – these are what give onions and garlic their pungent smell.

Scientists are still uncertain of how fruit and vegetables provide their health-boosting effects. Studies suggest that antioxidants play a vital role, by mopping up the harmful free radicals that damage the body's cells. Free radicals increase our risk of cancer, by damaging our DNA, and contribute to the atherosclerosis ('furred' arteries) that can lead to heart disease and stroke. So, by neutralising these damaging molecules, the antioxidants in food can help us to live longer, healthier lives.

But when researchers carried out clinical trials, giving people antioxidant pills, they didn't produce the expected health benefits. Why? It's not certain – but there seems to be something in the actual fruit and vegetables that the scientists haven't identified yet, or that just can't be put in a pill. One thing that's certain, though, is that eating the antioxidants in food form DOES work!

Get your five-a-day

We're recommended to eat five portions of fruit and vegetables a day – and more is better.

But what's a portion? Well, it's 80g, which is approximately equal to:

Fruit

- One medium apple
- 3 apricots
- 1 medium banana
- A handful of blackberries (about 8 to 10 berries)
- A handful of raspberries (about 15 to 20 berries)
- About 15 cherries
- 3 to 4 tablespoons of canned fruit in juice
- Half a large grapefruit
- A handful of grapes
- 1 medium peach or nectarine
- 1 medium pear
- Slice of melon (about 5cm)
- 2 kiwi fruit
- 2 satsumas, clementines or mandarins
- 1 large slice of fresh pineapple
- 2 medium plums
- About 8 strawberries

Vegetables

- 1 cereal bowlful of salad
- 1 large carrot
- 8 florets of broccoli
- 8 florets of cauliflower
- 8 Brussels sprouts
- 1 medium tomato
- 6 cherry tomatoes
- 8 spring onions (white plus green leaves)
- 1 medium onion
- 3 heaped tablespoons of peas
- 4 heaped tablespoons of runner beans

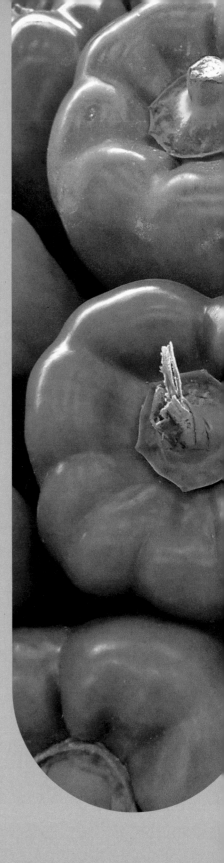

- Half a medium sweet pepper
- 3 sticks of celery
- 12 button mushrooms
- A 6cm chunk of cucumber
- Half a large courgette
- 4 heaped tablespoons of shredded cabbage or kale
- 10 radishes
- 5 asparagus spears
- 1 sweetcorn cob or 5 baby corn
- Half a medium aubergine
- 1 medium sweet potato

Other sources

You can also count these towards your five-a-day – but only once for each:
- 1 tablespoon of dried fruit
- 1 small (150ml) glass of pure fruit juice
- 1 small can of baked beans

Fresh, tinned or frozen?

It's best to get your five-a-day from freshly harvested fruit and vegetables – but this obviously isn't always, or even often, possible.

The vitamin content of fruit and vegetables begins to decline as soon as they're harvested, so by the time they begin to look sad and wizened, they only have a fraction of their nutrients.

This means that it pays to buy little and often, if you can. If you have a garden, resolve to put aside a plot for growing your own food.

And don't ignore frozen food – flash-freezing stops nutrient loss in its tracks.

Canned fruit and vegetables are less nutritious, but are a good standby to have in the store cupboard. Because they are boiled during canning, much of their soluble B vitamins and vitamin C dissolves into the canning liquid. Often, this is highly sugared or salted, which means that if you use the liquid (to get the vitamins), you get the sugar or salt as well. And if you throw it away, you lose the vitamins.

Note that potatoes don't count towards your five-a-day – they're classed as starchy foods instead.

Top tips
How to increase the fruit in your diet

Breakfast tips:

- Add fresh, tinned, stewed or dried fruit to muesli or breakfast cereal.

Main meal tips:

- Instead of a dessert, serve pieces of apple or pear, some grapes, and small slices of cheese.
- Make home-made pork burgers from lean minced pork, finely chopped onion and a grated apple.

Snack tips:

- Keep your fruit bowl topped up and in plain sight – you'll be more likely to eat from it.
- If you're travelling, take fruit as a healthy snack. You might find it more convenient (and easier for children) to pre-slice some fruits and carry them in a lidded container. Add a squeeze of lemon juice to apple and pears, to prevent them from discolouring.
- Make fruit smoothies from frozen berries, ice cubes and skimmed milk, or low-fat natural yogurt if you like a thicker texture.
- Keep a pot of dried fruit and unsalted nuts in your desk for when you get peckish at work.

Dessert tips:

- Purée fruit (add a tiny amount of honey if necessary). Put a scoop of low-fat quark (a soft cheese) on a plate, or some low-fat fromage frais or yogurt in a bowl, and drizzle the purée over.
- Slice some pineapple and banana, sprinkle over a little brown sugar, and grill or bake until the sugar melts. Keep your eye on it as the sugar burns easily and it could become bitter. Serve with a spoonful of low-fat natural fromage frais.
- Fill home-made pancakes with fruit or fruit purée.
- Make kebabs from chunks of fruit threaded onto skewers and lightly grill them. Try pineapple, pear, nectarine, mango and peach.
- Make low-sugar fruit crumbles with oaty toppings.

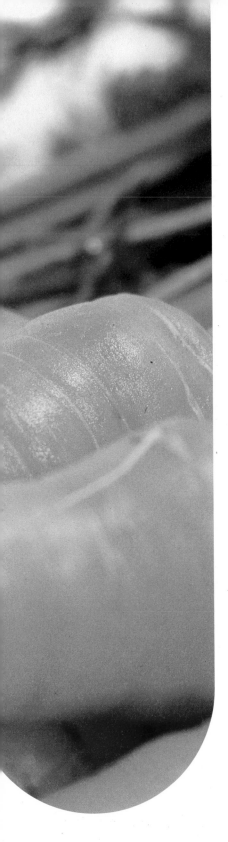

- Make a fruit fool from puréed mango and low-fat natural yogurt or fromage frais.
- Try baked apples, or pears poached in red grape juice, for dessert.

How to increase the vegetables in your diet

- For a quick meal, make an omelette and add thinly sliced mushroom (sautéed in a tiny quantity of olive oil) or some frozen vegetables, such as peppers, sweetcorn, broccoli or spinach.
- Make a tortilla (a thick Spanish omelette, served cut into wedges) adding wedges of fresh tomato.
- Make a stir-fry from vegetables such as finely sliced carrot, onion, courgette, mushroom, small sprigs of broccoli and bean sprouts, with chicken, turkey or prawns to provide protein. Add a splash of soy sauce and some Chinese five-spice powder for an Oriental taste.
- Up the veg in your pizza by adding baby spinach leaves, onion, tomatoes, peppers, mushrooms and sweetcorn.
- Toss a handful of cooked beans or crunchy sprouts on your salad. (Or, if you have a sweet tooth, increase your fruit by adding chopped apples, raisins or sliced dried unsulphured apricots.)
- Try veggie instead of meat lasagne.
- When making spaghetti Bolognese, reduce the amount of meat you use, and increase the amount of tinned tomato, and vegetables such as chopped onion and carrot, and sliced mushrooms. Or consider making a vegetarian version using lentils instead of meat, or half-and-half – you'll instantly cut the saturated fat and boost the fibre content.
- Add extra vegetables such as carrots, green beans and aubergine to your stews and casseroles.
- Find a vegetable soup recipe you like (try ours on page 151) and experiment! Throw in loads of different vegetables, whatever takes your fancy.
- Try our Chickpea Chilli on page 166 – it's packed with tasty vegetables.
- Cram as much salad – lettuce, tomato slices, onion, cucumber, mild baby spinach leaves – into your sandwiches, wraps and pitta pockets as you can.
- For packed lunches, or as an accompaniment to barbecue food or cold meats, make a rice or pasta salad, with a low-fat balsamic vinegar dressing and plenty of finely chopped spring onion, sweetcorn, finely chopped pepper and peas.

- When eating out, order salads, or boiled or steamed vegetables, as your side dishes, rather than chips.
- Snack on raw vegetables such as sticks of carrots, strips of celery, pepper or cucumber (seeds removed), or even sprigs of broccoli or cauliflower.

Shopping tips:

- Buy fruit and vegetables a little at a time, if you can, to avoid waste. Or buy fruit under-ripe and ripen it at home.
- Reduce the cost, and limit food air miles, by buying produce that can be grown in Britain, in season.

You'll find more on fabulous fruits in Chapter 8.

It's easy to get your five-a-day – or more

Here's an example of how you could tot up an impressive twelve portions of fruit and veg a day – without feeling that you're living on rabbit food!

Breakfast (3 portions of fruit):

A serving of porridge made with skimmed or semi-skimmed milk, topped with a chopped banana and a tablespoon of sultanas and sweetened with a teaspoon of honey, if needed. A small glass (110ml) of fresh fruit juice.

Snack (1 portion of vegetables):

A pot of veggie sticks (carrot, pepper, celery, cucumber, with healthy hummus (see recipe on page 178).

Lunch (2 portions of vegetables, 1 portion of fruit):

A pot of cottage cheese with pineapple with a bowl of salad leaves and a medium sliced tomato and 4 crispbreads. A handful of grapes.

Snack (1 portion of fruit):

An apple or a peach and a slice of malt loaf.

Dinner (3 portions of vegetables, 1 portion of fruit):

Butter bean and vegetable bake with green beans and broccoli. 3 stewed plums with fromage frais.

Total: 6 portions of fruit and 6 portions of vegetables, making a total of 12-a-day!

Research has shown that when people increase their fruit (and vegetable) intake, their intake of fat almost always falls, and they lose weight if they need to.

Get enough calcium

We all need calcium in our diets, for healthy bones – our skeleton contains about 1.5kg (3 pounds) of this vital mineral. Calcium also plays a role in nerve and muscle function.

Our needs are greatest at certain stages of our lives, namely:

- Childhood and adolescence (for bone growth)
- Your twenties (for building bone density)
- When breast-feeding (providing calcium for the baby in the breast milk)

Pregnant women need extra calcium to build the baby's bones, but the mother's body becomes super-efficient at absorbing the mineral from her diet during this time, so the actual requirement does not go up.

Most of the calcium in the UK diet comes from dairy products, such as milk, yogurt, fromage frais and cheese (including cottage cheese). The majority of us can get all the calcium we need from three portions of low-fat dairy products a day.

These could be:

- A medium (200ml) glass of skimmed or semi-skimmed milk
- A small pot (150ml) of low-fat natural yogurt or cottage cheese
- A small piece (30g, or matchbox-sized) of cheese

Don't worry if you're allergic or intolerant to dairy products – there are other good sources of calcium. Portion for portion, tofu and tinned sardines are far richer in calcium than milk! Other tinned fish where the bones are mashed into the fish and eaten (such as salmon), seeds such as sesame seeds, and some green vegetables are also good. Some soya milk is enriched with added calcium, but this varies widely between brands.

Here are some of the best calcium sources (per portion):

Dairy sources of calcium

	mg calcium
200ml glass milk (skimmed or semi-skimmed)	240mg
30g slice of cheese	222mg
150g pot of cottage cheese	191mg
150g low-fat yogurt	210mg

Non-dairy sources of calcium

	mg calcium
125g tin sardines	580mg
125g tin salmon	114mg
80g curly kale	120mg
80g spring greens	60mg
Small 220g tin red kidney beans	156mg
Small 200g tin baked beans	117mg
100g plain tofu	510mg
24g sesame seeds	134mg
1 slice wholemeal bread	90mg
30g dried figs	75mg
200ml glass soya milk	Approx 178mg

Vitamin D

In order to absorb and use calcium, our bodies need vitamin D, which is found in fish and dairy products. The action of sunlight on the skin also enables the body to make some of its own vitamin D. In the UK, about 20 minutes' daily exposure of the face and hands to the kind of sun we get during the spring and summer months is generally enough. However, because unfortunately this kind of sunshine isn't always easy to come by, we need to keep our bodies' levels topped up with vitamin D from our diets. Also, some groups of people, for example those with darker skin, or who cover up their skin for cultural reasons, or who are housebound, may not get enough vitamin D from sunlight alone.

Don't be tempted to think that because a little sunshine is good for you, more is better – the health risks of frying yourself in the sun far outweigh the benefits.

Calcium enemies

Some foods can hinder your absorption of calcium, or hasten its removal from your bones.

- **Caffeine** – there's some evidence that caffeine (such as that found in drinks like coffee, tea and cola) can increase the amount of calcium excreted from the body.
- **Fizzy drinks** – the phosphoric acid in carbonated cola drinks can decrease the uptake of calcium from food.
- **Fibre** – in large amounts fibre can hinder the absorption of calcium from food. However, a healthy balanced diet (like the eating plan in this book), containing plenty of fibre but not too much, won't compromise your ability to get enough calcium.
- **Tea** – tannins in tea bind with calcium in the gut, preventing it from being absorbed. Drink tea separately from meals, to avoid blocking the uptake of calcium from your food.

The recommended daily intake of calcium is 700mg for adults. Teenagers need more – 800mg for girls and 1,000mg for boys.

Top tips

Getting enough calcium:

- Have three portions of low-fat dairy products every day.
- Learn to love tofu – marinated, it's wonderful in stir-fries. And you can use soft (or silken) tofu in desserts.
- Have a tin of sardines or salmon every week – mash the bones into the fish and eat them.
- Make vegetarian chillies and stews with red kidney beans.
- Sprinkle sesame seeds on your cereal and on salads.
- Snack on dried figs.

Get enough iron

Iron is the mineral that's most commonly deficient in the diets of people in the developed world. We can store iron in our bodies, but once these iron stores are run down, we don't have enough iron to make the right amount of haemoglobin – the pigment in blood that is used to carry oxygen around the body. And if we don't have sufficient haemoglobin, we suffer the symptoms of iron-deficiency anaemia, including tiredness, weakness and lethargy. Children and adolescents suffering from anaemia will struggle in school, because they get tired easily and find it hard to concentrate. Many things conspire to put us at risk from iron deficiency. All of these can increase your risk of low iron levels.

High iron demands:
- Periods of rapid growth – for example childhood and adolescence
- Pregnancy
- Breast-feeding – iron is passed on to the baby in the milk
- Women who have heavy periods (iron is lost every month)

And these things hinder iron absorption:
- Drinks containing tannin and caffeine, such as tea and coffee – keep these for drinking between meals
- Foods that are very rich in fibre (however, this is only a problem in small children eating very-high-fibre diets, or adults whose fibre intake is way over the recommended amount of 18g per day)

We get iron from all kinds of sources, animal and vegetarian, and both kinds have advantages and disadvantages.

There are two sources of iron in our diet – animal and vegetarian.

Animal iron:
- Found in meat (especially red meat), poultry, fish and eggs
- Plus point – easier for our bodies to absorb than vegetarian iron
- Minus point – higher in fat (especially saturated fat) than vegetarian iron

Vegetarian iron:
- Found in beans and lentils, dried fruit (especially apricots), blackstrap molasses, some green leafy vegetables, and breakfast cereals which have been fortified with iron
- Plus point – lower in fat (especially saturated fat) and fibre than animal iron
- Minus point – much harder for the body to absorb than animal iron

Top tips

Upping your iron:

- Unless you're a vegetarian, have good-quality lean red meat once or twice a week. Buy organic if you can.
- Eat lean poultry, fish and eggs, as another good source of animal iron.
- A little bit of animal iron in a meal that contains vegetarian iron increases the uptake of the hard-to-absorb vegetarian iron. So, if you make a chilli con carne with lean mince and kidney beans, the meat will boost the absorption of the iron in the beans.
- Eat or drink something containing vitamin C (such as a glass of pure orange juice) when you have vegetarian iron (for example, beans, lentils or green leafy vegetables) in a meal. The vitamin C increases the amount of vegetarian iron you absorb. Red peppers are also excellent for vitamin C, so incorporate them into dishes containing vegetarian iron.

Other vitamins and minerals

Iron and calcium are important minerals that many people neglect in their diets. But what about all the other vitamins and minerals? We need them all, albeit in very small quantities, for a variety of reasons. For example, phosphorus helps make up the structure of our bones, while zinc supports the immune system. Many of the B vitamins act as 'spark plugs', setting off the reactions involved in metabolism. And the antioxidant vitamins, such as vitamins A, C and E, protect our cells by mopping up harmful free-radical molecules.

Vitamin	Function	Animal sources	Vegetarian sources
Vitamin A	Essential for vision; also needed for healthy skin and mucous membranes lining the mouth, eyelids, throat, digestive tract and vagina	These contain retinol, or 'pre-formed' vitamin A: Liver, meat, oily fish, dairy products, eggs	These contain betacarotene, which the body can convert into vitamin A: Green vegetables (spinach, cabbage, broccoli), and yellow and orange vegetables (carrots, sweet potatoes, apricots, peaches, cantaloupe melon)
B vitamins (vitamins B1, B2, B3, B5 and B6, plus B12 – see separate listing below)	Needed for the metabolism of energy from food	Meat, eggs, dairy products	Unrefined cereals and grains, beans and lentils, nuts, seeds, fortified breakfast cereals, green leafy vegetables such as spinach and watercress

Vitamin	Function	Animal sources	Vegetarian sources
Folic acid (folate)	Important during pregnancy and pre-conception, for reducing the risk of birth defects; helps the body to absorb nutrients effectively; supports the immune system; helps prevent a kind of anaemia	Liver, eggs	Brown rice, wheat germ, fortified breakfast cereals, pulses (beans and lentils), nuts, green leafy vegetables, broccoli, citrus fruit, apricots
Vitamin B12	Needed for the production of red blood cells	Red meat, fish, shellfish, eggs, dairy products	Not found in non-animal foods, but produced in small amounts by harmless bacteria in our gut
Vitamin C	Supports the immune system and acts as an antioxidant; required for wound healing; boosts absorption of iron from food		Fruit (especially kiwi fruit, blackcurrants, strawberries, citrus fruits), red and yellow peppers, tomatoes, Brussels sprouts
Vitamin D	Absorption of calcium, needed for healthy bones and teeth	Oily fish (e.g. salmon, trout, sardines, mackerel), meat, eggs, dairy products	Produced in the body by the action of sunlight on skin; it is also added to margarines and low-fat spreads, and fortified breakfast cereals
Vitamin E	Needed for a healthy reproductive system, and supporting the immune system; also important for nerves and muscles		Nuts and seeds and their oils, wholemeal bread, wheat germ, avocado, spinach, broccoli
Vitamin K	Needed for blood clotting after injury; required for healthy bones	Eggs, fish oils, dairy products	Green leafy vegetables; also produced in small amounts by harmless bacteria in the gut

Mineral	Function	Animal sources	Non-animal sources
Iron	Production of red blood cells; transport of oxygen around the body	Liver, kidney, red meat, chicken, eggs	Beans and lentils, green vegetables, dried fruit (especially apricots), fortified flour
Calcium	Building and maintaining healthy bones and teeth; nerve and muscle function	Dairy products, tinned fish where the bones are eaten (e.g. sardines and salmon)	Tofu, beans and lentils, sesame seeds, almonds, dried fruit (especially figs), kale and other green leafy vegetables, fortified flour
Phosphorus	Structural mineral found in the skeleton and teeth	Meat, fish, eggs, dairy products	Grains, seeds, beans and lentils, fruit and vegetables
Magnesium	Required for muscle function; needed for healthy bones; also involved in the body's response to stress	Meat, dairy products	Green vegetables, nuts and seeds, wholegrains, beans and lentils, dried fruits, mushrooms
Potassium	Controlling blood pressure; regulation of body fluids		Nuts (especially almonds and hazelnuts), sesame seeds, bananas, lentils, green leafy vegetables
Zinc	Required for a healthy immune system and preventing infection; needed for sperm formation in men	Oysters, meat, fish, shellfish, chicken, eggs, dairy products	Seeds (especially pumpkin seeds), nuts, wholegrains, green leafy vegetables, pulses
Selenium	Supporting the immune system	Meat, liver and kidney, fish, seafood, eggs	Brazil nuts, sesame seeds

Don't worry – you don't need to learn all of the vitamins and minerals and what they do. If you eat a balanced diet, with plenty of variety, such as the eating plan in this book, you'll get all you need (unless you have special requirements – see 'Are supplements the answer?').

Are supplements the answer?

Many people are tempted to pop a vitamin or mineral supplement to make up for their unhealthy eating habits.

Supplements should never be seen as a quick fix for a poor diet. It's no use living on junk food, then just taking a pill and thinking you'll be fine!

Also, some people think that if vitamins and minerals are good for you, then taking a 'mega-dose' must be even better. Impressive-sounding health claims have been made for high-dose supplements, such as their potential to reduce the risk of cancer and heart disease. However, the evidence for these nutrients reducing our disease risk is seen when we get them from food, not from pills. As yet there's no conclusive evidence that the pills help at all, and they could even be dangerous. Some vitamins and minerals, notably the fat-soluble vitamins A, D, E and K, can accumulate in the body to toxic levels.

Some sections of the population, who have particularly high nutrient requirements or who find it impossible to get enough from a normal healthy diet, might benefit from a good-quality low-dose multivitamin and mineral supplement. Low dose means no more than the recommended daily intake, to top up their natural levels. For example, pregnant women, those planning a baby, children and the elderly have higher nutrient needs, so might be advised to take a low-dose supplement. In these cases, look for a supplement that's specially formulated for your particular age group or life stage, such as pregnancy. Smokers have an increased requirement for vitamin C, so might like to take a vitamin C supplement (not a mega-dose) as well as eating plenty of C-rich fruit and vegetables. If you're unsure whether you have special nutritional needs, ask your doctor, practice nurse, or a dietician or registered nutritionist.

The bottom line is: supplements should only ever be used as a supplement to a healthy diet, not as a replacement for one!

Good fats

Fats have gained a bad reputation, demonised as being the culprit behind obesity and clogging up our arteries. It's true that too much fat, especially if it's the wrong kind of fat (the saturated and trans fats you'll meet on page 60), can cause us to pile on the pounds, and contribute to atherosclerosis ('furring' or clogging of the arteries). But it's wrong to be fat-phobic.

Fats are an essential part of our diet. Some vitamins, such as A, D, E and K, are only found in fat-containing foods. Fats make up 25 to 35 per cent of a healthy woman's body, and 15 to 25 per cent of a healthy man's, and much of our brains and cell membranes are composed of healthy fats. A small amount of fat is needed to protect our internal organs, and certain fats are also required for our bodies to make particular hormones.

What about cholesterol? The two kinds

In order to understand why there are 'good fats' and 'bad fats', it helps to understand a bit about cholesterol.

There are two kinds of cholesterol found in the bloodstream. One – LDL cholesterol – is harmful, as it increases your risk of atherosclerosis and therefore heart disease and stroke. The other – HDL cholesterol – is good for you, as it removes fats from your blood, decreasing your risk of clogged arteries.

We need to do and eat things that lower our levels of 'bad' LDL cholesterol, and raise our levels of 'good' HDL cholesterol.

It's easy:

- Eat moderate amount of unsaturated fats
- Cut down saturated and trans fats
- Maintain a healthy weight
- Keep active – take plenty of exercise

We need a moderate amount of the 'good' fats to keep our bodies and brains in tiptop condition. These are the unsaturated fats, which can be divided into monounsaturated and polyunsaturated fats.

Monounsaturated fats

These fats are good for our cholesterol levels. Oils rich in monounsaturated fats include olive oil, canola oil and peanut oil. When you need a small amount of oil for frying, olive and canola are the best to use, as they are less susceptible to being damaged by heat and forming harmful free-radical molecules. Nuts and seeds also contain monounsaturates. Macadamia nuts are excellent, as are almonds and pistachios. The oil found in avocados is also monounsaturated.

Polyunsaturated fats

These also benefit cholesterol levels, though not so much as monounsaturates. Safflower oil, sunflower oil and corn oil are all good sources of polyunsaturates. Omega-3 and omega-6 fatty acids are subgroups of polyunsaturates, found in oily fish, nuts and seeds. They help lower our cholesterol levels, reduce our risk of heart disease, and even benefit our mood.

Omega-3 fatty acids

These are found mainly in oily fish, such as salmon, trout, fresh tuna, mackerel and sardines. They're also found in certain plant oils, especially flaxseed (linseeds), but the body has to convert the omega-3 from these vegetarian sources to the active form it needs, so fish is far better if you are able to eat it. The omega-3s in oily fish are directly useable by the body.

Omega-3s are fantastic for cardiovascular health (the heart and blood vessels). They are also good for our cholesterol levels, as well as making the blood less 'sticky' and therefore less likely to form life-threatening clots.

Omega-3s are also good for the brain – both in building its structure and ensuring its proper function. Research has shown that people in countries with a high omega-3 intake are less likely to suffer from depression, or from dementia in old age. Studies are also suggesting that omega-3s can actually help to treat depression and even produce dramatic benefits in children suffering from ADHD (attention deficit hyperactivity disorder). It certainly seems likely that these healthy oils could help keep anyone's moods calm and stable. Perhaps fish's reputation as 'brain food' isn't an old wives' tale after all!

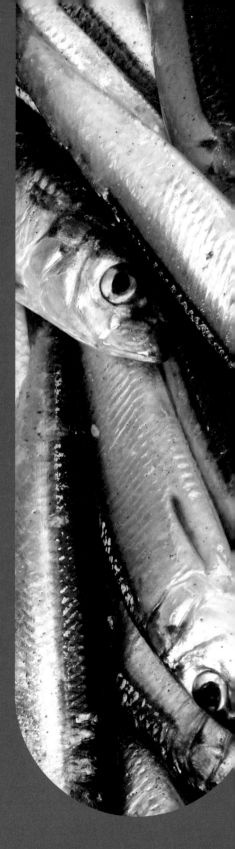

Omega-6 fatty acids

These healthy oils have similar heart health benefits to omega-3s, but the effects aren't quite so dramatic. They may also reduce our risk of type-2 diabetes, and reduce the symptoms of asthma and eczema.

Omega-6s are found in nuts and seeds, as well as some vegetable oils, including corn oil, sunflower oil and safflower oil.

Top tips
Increasing the good fats in your diet:
- Eat oily fish at least once a week (but see 'Oily fish and pollutants')
- Use a low-fat olive spread that's high in monounsaturates and free from hydrogenated (trans) fats on your toast and sandwiches
- When you do fry (for example to stir-fry) use small amounts of canola or olive oil, and use olive oil in salads
- Add avocado to salads and sandwiches, or make guacamole to accompany a low-fat Mexican dish
- Sprinkle ground linseeds, or other seeds, on your cereal
- Eat unsalted nuts and seeds as a snack
- Remember, though, that all fats are high in calories, so can cause you to put on weight, so go easy on the portion sizes

Oily fish and pollutants

Some oily fish can contain low levels of pollutants, which can build up to higher levels in the body over time if you eat them often. Because of this, pregnant women and those planning a baby shouldn't eat oily fish more than twice a week, and shouldn't eat swordfish, marlin or shark at all. This is because they can contain low levels of heavy-metal toxins such as mercury, which although they probably wouldn't harm the mother, could damage the baby.

But pregnant women should still aim for one or two portions of fish per week, one of which should be oily fish, because the omega-3s in oily fish are needed for healthy brain development in babies. They might also like to talk with their doctor about taking a supplement for pregnant women that contains omega-3s.

None of us should be put off oily fish. The health benefits of eating it far outweigh any tiny potential risk.

Getting enough fibre

Fibre doesn't have a very exciting reputation – roughage, bowels and bran aren't exactly sexy subjects!

And, sad to say, many of us don't eat enough fibre – we should be getting 18g a day, but the average intake in the UK is a mere 12g.

Getting plenty of fibre can:

- Help balance blood-sugar and energy levels
- Reduce the risk of digestive problems such as constipation and IBS (irritable bowel syndrome)
- Help you to maintain your weight, or lose weight if you need to, by filling you up
- Encourage the growth of beneficial 'friendly bacteria' in the gut
- Reduce the risk of certain cancers
- Benefit your cholesterol levels
- Reduce the risk of heart disease and stroke

There are two kinds of fibre, with different health benefits.

Insoluble fibre is the kind we used to call 'roughage', and it's good for digestive health. It 'bulks out' the contents of the digestive system, smoothing the contents of the gut on its way, and helping to prevent constipation and IBS. By keeping the gut contents moving, it reduces the amount of time any potentially dangerous substances are in contact with the bowel wall, reducing the risk of bowel cancer.

Good sources of insoluble fibre include wholegrains, vegetables and fruit (especially the skins), and beans and pulses.

Soluble fibre is a 'gluey' kind of fibre – it's what makes porridge sticky. Soluble fibre reduces the impact that foods containing sugar have on your blood-sugar levels, helping to keep your blood-sugar levels stable. This is particularly important for those whose blood-sugar control isn't so good, such as 'borderline diabetics' or 'pre-diabetics'.

Soluble fibre also lowers the levels of harmful LDL cholesterol in the blood, therefore reducing our risk of clogged arteries, heart disease and strokes. It also promotes the growth of the 'friendly bacteria' that inhabit the large intestine.

The main sources of soluble fibre are oats, beans and lentils, but fruit and vegetables are also good sources.

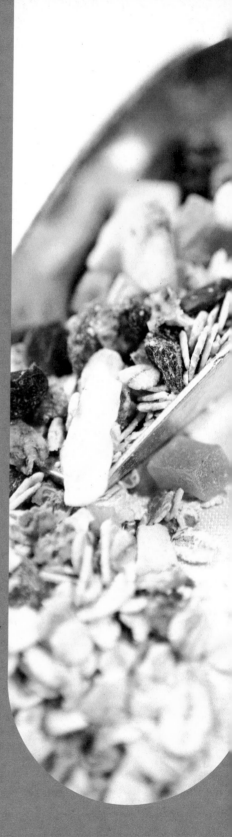

Reasons to eat wholegrains

Wholegrains include the 'brown' or natural versions of starchy carbohydrates, such as brown rice, wholemeal pasta, wholemeal bread, wholemeal noodles, oats, buckwheat, millet and brown couscous. Wholegrains help in all sorts of ways:

- High in gut-healthy insoluble fibre; some kinds (especially oats) are rich in heart-healthy soluble fibre
- Low in fat (and the fat they do contain is the healthy unsaturated kind)
- A good source of many vitamins, especially the B vitamins and vitamin E
- Rich in trace minerals, such as antioxidant and immune-boosting selenium
- Contain antioxidant polyphenols
- Contain phyto-oestrogens, which may act as oestrogen-boosters if your oestrogen level is low, and oestrogen-dampeners if your oestrogen level is high
- Can help keep your blood-sugar levels smooth and consistent
- Help prevent constipation
- Help you feel sustained between meals, so it's easier to lose weight or maintain a healthy weight
- Can reduce your risk of cancer
- Can reduce your risk of cardiovascular disease (heart disease and stroke)
- Can reduce your risk of type-2 diabetes

Top tips

Get enough fibre:

- Go wholegrain – switch to wholemeal bread, brown pasta, brown rice, and try other wholegrains such as buckwheat, millet and quinoa
- Eat more fruit and vegetables, preferably with their skins (buy organic when possible)
- Replace some of the meat in your diet with beans and lentils
- Snack on high-fibre foods such as fruit, vegetable sticks, nuts and seeds
- Make more of your food from scratch – processed foods are generally lower in fibre than 'real' food prepared at home

Keeping hydrated

Our bodies are 50 to 75 per cent water. Without food, people can survive for six weeks, but without water we would die within a few days.

Dehydration doesn't just make you feel rough – in the long run it can contribute to dry skin, constipation and kidney stones.

Do you drink enough water? Even mild dehydration can make you feel weak, lethargic and dizzy, or give you a headache. Don't wait until you feel thirsty before you have a drink of water – thirst is a signal that your body is already well on the way to dehydration, so it's important to drink before your thirst demands, and to keep your fluid levels topped up throughout the day. Children and the elderly aren't very good at responding to their 'thirst signals', so it's important to encourage them to drink enough water.

You should drink one and a half to two litres of water per day – that's about eight to ten medium-sized glasses. You can get some of this from your food, particularly fresh, juicy foods like fruits and vegetables, but you'll need to get most of it from fluids, preferably pure water.

Herb and fruit teas, and diluted fruit juice, count towards your fluid intake as well. Tea and coffee also count, even though caffeine is a diuretic, so increases the rate of fluid loss from your body. The water content of the drink more than offsets this; you just need to remember it's not as hydrating as herb and fruit teas or water.

Milk has a high fluid content, but it's more of a 'snack' than a thirst quencher.

Fizzy drinks and squashes should be avoided because of the sugars and artificial chemicals they contain. And alcohol certainly doesn't count when you're trying to reach your fluid target.

Beware the calories, fat and sugar contained in many drinks. Drinks don't fill you up as much as food – even if they contain exactly the same number of calories – so it's easy to put on weight without realising why. A hot chocolate from a trendy coffee bar can contain more fat, sugar and calories than a meal!

Here are some of the main liquid calorie offenders:

Drink	Calories	Sugar Equivalent	Fat Content
Thick milkshake (medium, fast-food restaurant):	390kcal	13tsp	10g
Hot chocolate (medium, full fat milk):	448kcal	13tsp	24g
Full fat latte (medium):	265kcal	0tsp	14g
Full fat cappuccino (medium):	153kcal	0tsp	8g
Fizzy drink (medium, fast food restaurant):	170kcal	8tsp	0g

For a list of calorie counts for alcohol, see page 73.

Top tips
Stay hydrated:
- Start as you mean to go on – drink a glass of water first thing in the morning.
- Buy a two-litre bottle of mineral water, and keep refilling your glass, or using it to make hot drinks, throughout the day. You need to get through the whole bottle by bedtime. If you don't want to keep buying bottled water, refill the bottle from the tap the next day.
- Keep a glass of water beside you throughout the day, and keep sipping from it. Drink little and often.
- Carry a small water bottle when you're out and about.
- If you're not used to drinking much water, work up to your target gradually, to allow your body to adjust. Otherwise it could make you feel dizzy and give you headaches.

Exercise and Activity

Even if you eat the best diet in the world, you won't reap all the benefits if you don't get enough exercise.

Being physically active can:

- Improve your energy levels and stamina
- Help you to lose weight, if you need to, when combined with a healthy diet
- Lower your proportion of body fat, and increase your proportion of muscle; this has the added bonus of boosting your metabolic rate
- Reduce your risk of heart disease, by lowering your blood pressure and level of harmful LDL cholesterol
- Reduce your risk of certain types of cancer
- Reduce your risk of type-2 diabetes
- Some types of exercise (weight-bearing exercises) improve bone density, reducing your risk of osteoporosis
- Help to boost your mood; exercise stimulates the release of endorphins in the brain – these 'happy chemicals' produce a feeling of exhilaration and wellbeing
- Promote better sleep
- Improve your quality of life, encouraging you to 'get out and about', particularly later in life

Don't be daunted by exercise. It isn't all about scarily fit Amazons pounding the pavements at 5 a.m. every morning, willowy waifs tying themselves into pretzel-shapes at yoga classes, or beefy musclemen lifting huge weights. It's about people like YOU.

When you first start out, you don't have to do it for long, and it doesn't have to be exhausting. All you need to do is push your body a little further than it's used to, and make it work a little harder. Any more than that can be counterproductive, making you feel worn out and discouraged, and risking injury.

Only a third of men and a quarter of women in the UK are meeting the government targets for physical activity. We're supposed to take thirty minutes of moderate exercise five times a week, while children and young people should take sixty minutes.

As you get fitter, it'll get easier, and you'll have to do a little more in order to tax yourself. Soon you won't believe how unfit you used to be, and you'll be feeling the benefits.

Home, gym or outdoors – it's up to you.

Exercising at home

There are a huge variety of exercises you can do in the comfort of your own home. Why not buy an exercise DVD? Or invest in a good-quality treadmill, exercise bike, rowing machine or cross-trainer? If you haven't got that much money to spend, you can buy small dumbbells, wrist and ankle weights, and resistance bands for strength training. Or tone your tummy with a Hula Hoop. A skipping rope is great for aerobic fitness and co-ordination, and some home exercises don't need any equipment, such as press-ups, crunches, squats and leg lifts.

Home exercise plus points:
- Zero travel time, so it's convenient, and good for busy people
- Non-threatening – good if you're shy or self-conscious
- No membership fees

Home exercise minus points:
- Requires self-discipline
- Can be lonely
- No one-to-one expert help and encouragement

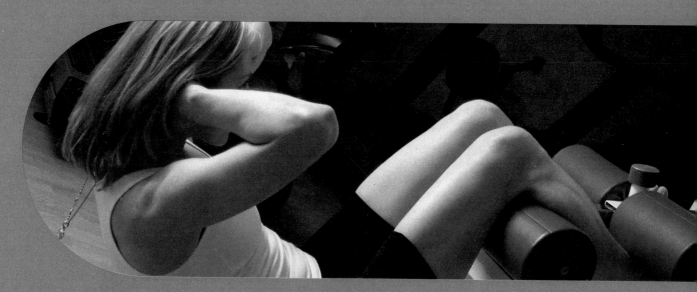

Exercising at the gym

If you're a social animal, you'll probably enjoy working out at a gym, or joining some exercise classes. An advantage of this is that you will have the encouragement of like-minded people, plus skilled instructors on hand. Gyms will also have the kind of high-tech equipment most of us could only dream of using at home. However, gyms can be expensive (especially if you decide they're not for you, when you've already forked out for your membership) and unless you're fortunate enough to have one at your workplace, you have to factor in the time and money spent getting there.

Gym plus points:
- More high-tech equipment available
- Social – make new friends and receive encouragement
- Experts on hand to offer advice

Gym minus points:
- You need to factor in your travelling time – this can make exercise inconvenient and you may be less likely to stick at it
- Membership fees can be expensive
- New exercisers can find the gym atmosphere intimidating rather than encouraging; visit a gym a few times before joining to decide whether it's for you

Exercising outdoors

Some of the best exercises involve getting out of doors – try walking, jogging, running, cycling, roller-blading, horse-riding or orienteering.

Outdoor exercise plus points:
- Often there's no travel time (for example, taking a walk around your local neighbourhood)
- Gets you out into the fresh air
- Generally doesn't require much specialist equipment

Outdoor exercise minus points:
- The British climate can be unpredictable and sometimes rather miserable; you'll need warm and waterproof clothing – or a fall-back plan for another form of exercise when the weather is too awful

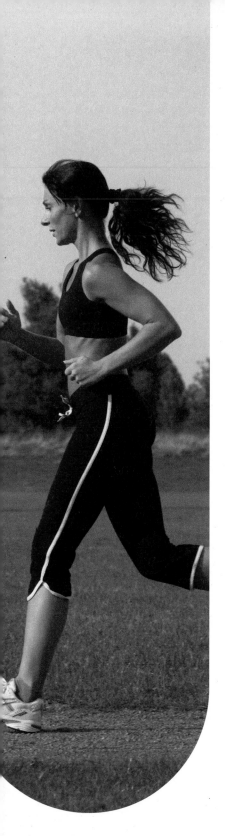

Sports

Consider joining a local sports club – most are very welcoming towards beginners, and because everyone's an enthusiast, you'll have plenty of encouragement. Try athletics, tennis, badminton, squash, netball, football, rugby or cricket.

More unusual exercises

Look out for adverts for classes and clubs in your local newspaper or library. Many schools make use of their large sports halls by running after-school and weekend classes. Try fencing, dancing (such as belly dancing, hip-hop, salsa or tango), Tai Chi, Pilates, yoga or kick boxing.

Don't be discouraged by the fact that there may be lots of people out there who are fitter than you, with better physiques than you. Don't be put off joining a gym or an exercise class just because everyone seems to be slim and gorgeous. Even if you feel like an ugly duckling in a pond full of swans, reassure yourself with the fact that the workout is doing you more good than it is them, and even they had to start somewhere.

In Chapter 1, we introduced the three kinds of fitness:

- Cardiovascular or aerobic fitness
- Strength or resistance fitness
- Flexibility fitness

They're all important, and you need to fit them all into your week. But it needn't take up all your free time, or put a lid on your social life. You don't have to spend a fortune either.

People come in different shapes, sizes and personalities, and all of these factors affect the kinds of activities that you'll be best at, and enjoy most. There's no such thing as a 'best' exercise – the best plan is the one you enjoy enough to stick to! Make sure you include a mixture of aerobic, strength and flexibility exercise.

And if you simply can't stand the idea of gyms and classes, then that's fine. Gyms and classes can be great for getting and keeping you motivated – a lot of people like the social aspect, and find it helpful to have a routine. But if that's not you, you can get all the exercise you need from simple activities like walking, jogging, cycling and swimming.

Aerobic exercise

Aerobic exercise is also called cardiovascular exercise, or 'cardio'. This is the kind of exercise that gets you breathing deeply and your heart pumping powerfully.

We need aerobic fitness to keep our hearts and lungs strong. The heart is a muscle and, like every other muscle, it gets stronger when it has to work harder. Exercising muscles need more oxygen, and aerobic exercise makes your heart beat faster and stronger, to pump more blood around the body.

And as your heart gets stronger, it doesn't have to work so hard when you're resting – this is why your resting heart rate will generally fall as you begin to feel the benefits of your exercise programme.

Aerobic exercise:

- Reduces your risk of heart attacks and stroke
- Burns calories and fat (helping you to lose weight)
- Builds stamina
- Increases your lung capacity and lung efficiency, so you don't get out of breath running up stairs
- Improves the muscle tone of the part of the body you're working
- Makes you feel good and relieves stress – aerobic exercise is the best kind of exercise to stimulate the release of serotonin, a brain chemical that makes you feel happy and contented

Good examples of aerobic exercise include:

- Brisk walking
- Jogging
- Running
- Cycling
- Swimming
- Trampolining
- Skipping
- Exercise machines such as treadmills, rowing machines, steppers, elliptical trainers
- Some sports (such as tennis, squash and badminton – depending on how much running around you do!)

In order to gain real benefits, you need to exercise to a level that makes you out of breath, for at least twenty minutes.

Strength exercise

Strength exercise is also known as resistance training or weight training. But don't let that put you off – it doesn't necessarily involve lifting weights.

This kind of exercise builds up the strength of your muscles. It won't turn you into a muscle-bound hulk, it will just give you that toned physique that will make clothes fit better and give you the confidence to wear what you like on the beach.

Strength training:
- Increases the strength of your muscles, so jobs like lifting and carrying things becomes easier
- Increases your ratio of body muscle to fat, meaning that you burn more calories even when you're resting
- Gives you a lithe, toned physique
- Lessens your risk of injury during exercise
- Slows down the natural muscle loss that occurs as you age

You strengthen your muscles by making them work against resistance, which is in the form of some kind of weight. This could be provided by hand-held dumb-bells or weights machines at a gym. You could even use your own bodyweight to provide resistance – push-ups, pull-ups from a bar, and sit-ups or crunches, are all forms of strength exercises.

Good forms of strength exercise include:
- Free weights – dumbbells you can use at the gym or buy to use at home
- Weights machines at the gym
- Exercises using gym balls
- Press-ups and pull-ups
- Squats and lunges
- Crunches or sit-ups
- Resistance bands

It's a good idea to do strength exercises about three or four times a week, aiming eventually for sessions of forty minutes to an hour each time. As you'll need to work all of your muscles over the week, it's a good idea to visit a gym for a few sessions and get some advice on putting together a routine, even if you don't intend to attend regularly. Alternatively you could buy a good book or DVD on resistance or strength training.

Flexibility

Flexibility exercises have a fantastic feel-good factor. Not only will they make everyday tasks like tying your shoelaces easier, they're also great for improving your balance and co-ordination, relieving stress and helping you to relax. Probably the best-known flexibility exercises are yoga and Pilates.

Yoga

There are many books, videos and DVDs available on yoga. They give you the opportunity to try it out without much cost, but there's also the disadvantage of not having anyone to tell you if you're doing it wrong. And if you're stretching or bending too far, you could injure yourself. If you are a complete novice, it's probably best to learn the techniques at a local class, where you'll also be able to meet other yoga enthusiasts.

Pilates

Pilates is considered one of the safest exercise techniques there is. It's a scientifically devised concept based on a thorough knowledge of the human body that works on the deep-core stability muscles, gradually strengthening them without stressing the joints or the heart. Movements are precise, controlled and continuous. It's often used by athletes and dancers regaining their fitness after an injury, but it has also gained a reputation for building a lean and lithe physique, a flat tummy and a dancer's posture.

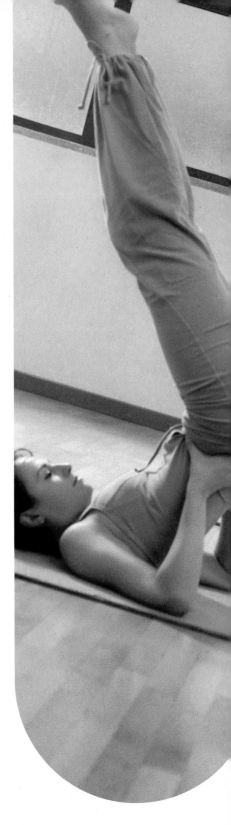

Getting started with exercise

Start off gently, say, with a brisk ten-minute walk every day. Once that's easy, add five minutes more for the next week. When you can easily walk for twenty minutes briskly, cut your walking back to four days a week, but on those days work on increasing the time you walk for until you can comfortably manage fifty minutes to an hour. As you get fitter, you could swap some of your walks for other aerobic exercises such as a cycle ride or swimming, or break into a jog for a couple of minutes every now and then during your walk – adjust the length of your session according to what you can manage.

You also need to schedule some exercise into the other days of the week. How about some strength training on two to four days, some flexibility exercises on one more, and a day off? You could also make some days 'multi-purpose', for example doing thirty minutes of aerobic exercise and fifteen minutes of resistance training.

Now you've devised your own exercise programme! You could also follow the example in our eight-week plan.

Warm up and cool down

Don't forget to warm up before you exercise, and cool down afterwards, to lessen your risk of pulling a muscle. Just do five minutes of walking (or a gentler version of the exercise you were planning to do, if it was something like cycling or swimming), before and afterwards. Give your main muscle groups a stretch, too.

Hidden exercise

You can increase your physical activity levels by sneaking 'exercise' into your everyday life. Try some of these:

- Leave the car at home, and walk or cycle wherever possible
- Get off the bus a stop earlier, or park further away from work or the shops, and walk the rest of the way
- Walk the children to school
- Take them to play football or Frisbee in the park – it will do you all good
- Cycle to work
- Take the stairs at work or when shopping, instead of the lift or escalator
- When you're at home and something needs to be taken upstairs, do it straight away, rather than leaving it on the bottom stair until there's a pile to take
- If you have a hands-free phone, walk about while you're talking
- If you have an exercise bike or treadmill, put it in your bedroom or somewhere you have a TV – then you can combine viewing with exercise
- Go for a walk at lunchtime, rather than staying at your desk
- When you're doing the housework, give it a little extra 'oomph' – introduce a few lunges when you're doing the vacuuming
- Get gardening – it can be surprisingly strenuous

Top tips

Getting active:

- Make it a habit – schedule regular exercise into your daily routine
- Set yourself goals – both long and short term
- Break your exercise into manageable chunks – it can be much less daunting than the thought of a long workout
- Sneak more activity into your day
- Concentrate on the forms of exercise that you enjoy – but don't be afraid to try something new
- Get the right gear – you don't have to spend a fortune on fancy outfits, but make sure that you have the right footwear and any necessary protective equipment (and wear something that makes you feel good about yourself!)
- Find an 'exercise buddy' – most people find that exercising with someone else provides motivation and encouragement
- Have a 'contingency plan' for when something prevents you from doing your usual exercise; for example, have something like a treadmill or exercise DVD that you can do at home, if you can't go for your usual swimming session, gym class or cycle ride

Safety first

If you have a health problem (if you're very overweight, have a heart problem, diabetes or joint problems), or if you're a smoker, ask your doctor before beginning an exercise programme. In fact, if you're at all worried if it's safe for you to exercise, check with your GP first. And remember:

- You shouldn't exercise when you've got a cold or flu
- You should always stop if you feel dizzy, or your heart is pounding alarmingly (this means you're exercising too vigorously)

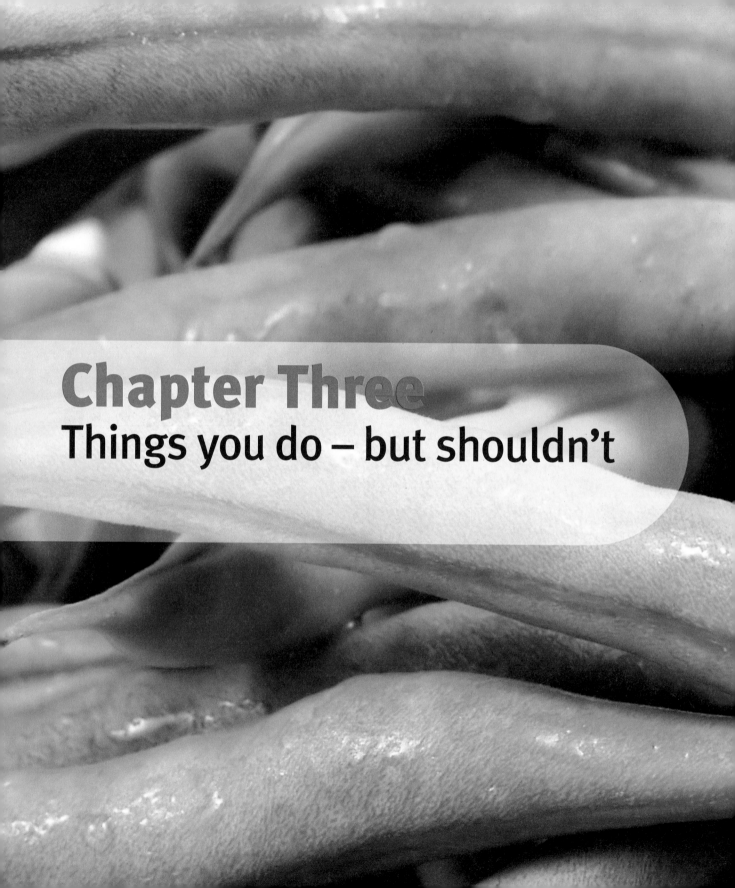

Chapter Three
Things you do – but shouldn't

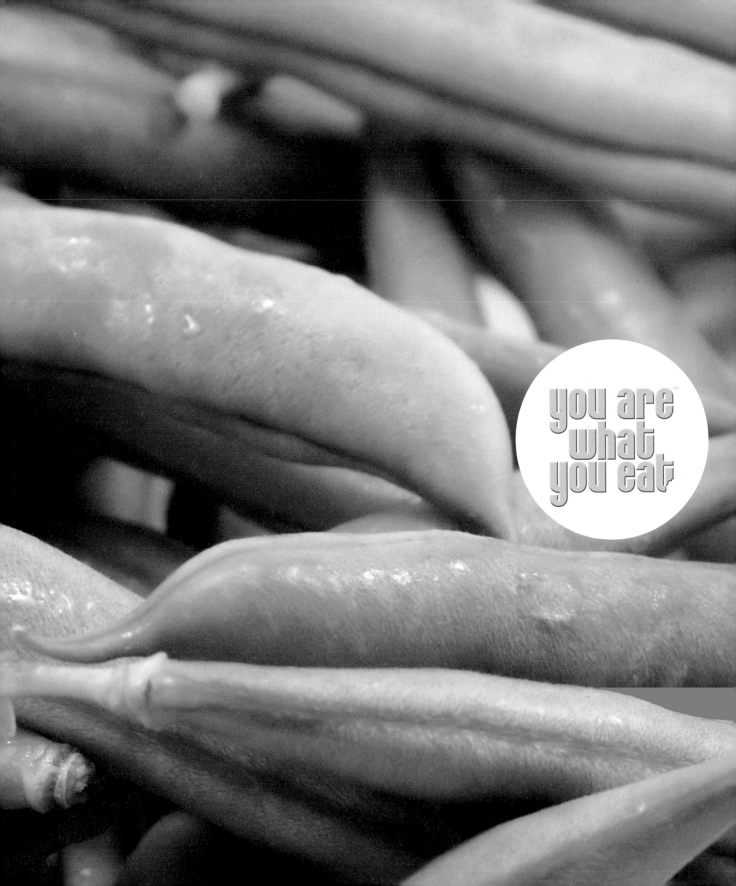

you are what you eat™

Nutritional Bugbears

We all have our own nutritional weaknesses, whether it's a fondness for biscuits or a love of greasy fried breakfasts. You may have a whole list of things you eat, but know you shouldn't.

And some of the things that are bad for us – especially if we eat them often or in large quantities – aren't immediately obvious.

We'll lead you through the minefield of nutritional nasties that sap your energy, increase your risk of illness, and crowd out the healthier ingredients from your diet.

The Bad Fats

Too much fat in our diet is bad news. For a start, fat is the food component that contains the most calories (more than protein and carbohydrate), so if we eat too much, we put on weight – with all the problems and health risks that brings.

The recommended maximum fat intake is for us to get no more than 35 per cent of our calories from fat (cautious nutritionists would say that 30 per cent is a better level).

Recommended maximum total daily fat intake:
- For an average man – 99g
- For an average woman – 75g

Remember this isn't just the butter or margarine you spread on your toast, and the oil you use for frying. Fat is concealed in even lean-looking meat, in eggs, milk and other dairy products, in salad dressings and sauces, as well as a vast array of manufactured foods.

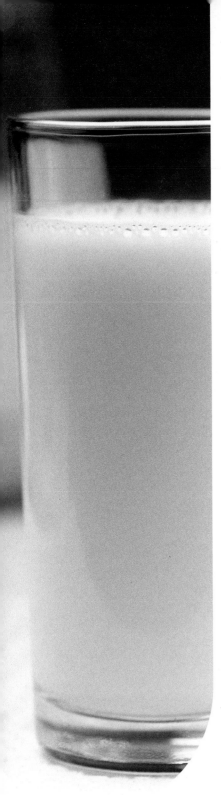

Fat-reducing swaps

High fat	Lower fat
Red meats (e.g. beef, lamb)	White meats (chicken, turkey)
Fatty poultry (duck, goose)	Low-fat poultry (chicken, turkey)
Processed meat products (sausages, pies)	Real cuts and joints of meat
Meals based around meat products	Meals based around beans and lentils
Curries	Tandoori and tikka dishes
Creamy pasta sauces	Tomato-based pasta sauces
Puff, flaky and short-crust pastry	Filo pastry
Fried chips	Home-made oven chips (see recipe on page 170)
Crisps	Baked bagel crisps
Full-fat milk	Skimmed or semi-skimmed milk
Full-fat, luxury or Greek yogurt	Low-fat or fat-free yogurt
Full-fat cream cheese	Low-fat soft cheese or cottage cheese
Full-fat mascarpone	Low-fat quark
Cheddar, Cheshire, Stilton, Roquefort	Feta, Camembert, Edam, Brie, mozzarella
Cream with desserts	Natural yogurt, quark or fromage frais
Ice cream	Frozen yogurt

What's the problem with fat?

Too much fat (and especially certain kinds of fat) is associated with:

- Obesity
- High cholesterol levels
- Heart disease
- Diabetes
- Stroke
- Certain kinds of cancer, including breast cancer and colon cancer

Although we need some of the healthy fats, we need to keep our total fat intake at a sensible level, and minimise our intake of the unhealthy fats.

There are two main kinds of unhealthy fats – saturated fats and trans fats.

Saturated fats

Characteristics of saturated fats:

- Generally found in animal products (meat, poultry, eggs, dairy products)
- Normally solid at room temperature – think of butter and lard, and the fat you find on meat (much of the fat in milk is saturated, but it's suspended in tiny droplets in the liquid)

Vegetable oils are generally better for us than animal fats, but you can also find saturated fats in certain plant products. Some of the oils from tropical plants are actually solid at room temperature, thanks to their high saturated-fat content. These include palm oil (found in lots of processed foods) and coconut oil.

If you're reading an ingredients list on a food label, and you see 'vegetable fat' – beware! It's likely to come from a tropical oil that is high in unhealthy saturated fat.

Recommended maximum daily intakes of saturated fat

Average woman – 21g
Average man – 28g

Six out of every seven people in the UK eat too much saturated fat.

Top tips

Cutting the saturated fat in your diet:

- When you're shopping at the supermarket, look for foods with a green 'traffic light label' for fat and saturated fat
- Trim the visible fat from meat
- Keep red meat to a maximum of two servings per week; red meat is higher in saturated fat than other meats
- Remove the fat from chicken and turkey – this is where most of the fat lurks
- Avoid processed meat products such as sausages, burgers and meat pies – they often use poor-quality fatty meat.
- You can buy low-fat burgers but check the label carefully as 'lower fat' burgers often still contain significant amounts.
- Replace meat protein with vegetarian protein, such as beans, lentils, etc. – these are almost saturated fat-free.

- Ban lard and suet from your house
- Instead of butter, use a low-fat spread that's high in monounsaturates (such as olive spread), in small quantities
- If you're making sandwiches with moist fillings, you won't need any spread
- Switch to low-fat versions of dairy products: skimmed milk, low-fat yogurt and fromage frais, low-fat soft cheese, and low-fat or half-fat cheese
- Beware cheesy toppings – a generous serving of cheese packs a hefty dose of saturated fat
- Use tasty cheeses like vintage Cheddar or Parmesan – the stronger taste means you don't have to use so much

Trans fats

Fortunately, many brands and restaurants are removing trans fats from their products, and a lot of supermarkets are taking them out of their own-label foods.

These unhealthy fats contribute to the same kind of health problems as saturated fats – they can lead to weight gain, clog your arteries and increase your risk of heart disease and stroke. But they're probably even worse for you than saturated fats. Because they're very similar in structure to 'healthy fats' – the oils you read about in the previous chapter – the body can mistakenly use them instead of their healthier counterparts. And a body that uses trans fats as fuel and in it's cell structure doesn't function as well as one that runs on healthy fats.

The main sources of trans fats in our diets are the hydrogenated or partially hydrogenated fats found in processed foods, and which are used for frying in some fast-food restaurants.

Both kinds of hydrogenated fats are unsaturated fats that have been altered by the food industry to give them different properties. They're cheap, and they give foods a longer shelf life.

Hydrogenated fats (and therefore trans fats) find their way into a huge proportion of processed foods. You'll find them in ready-meals, sauces in jars and packets, instant drinks and instant soups, cakes and cake mixes, biscuits, pastries, sweets, desserts, pudding mixes, some ice creams, chocolates and chocolate bars.

Top tips

Cutting the trans fats in your diet:

- Minimise your intake of processed foods – these are the main source of trans fats in our diets; make as much of your food as possible from scratch
- Don't eat fast food – it's often fried in hydrogenated oils
- Read the labels – look for 'trans fat free', and avoid anything with 'hydrogenated' on the ingredients list

What about cholesterol?

'Cholesterol is bad for you' – right? Well, only if it's the wrong kind of cholesterol.

It's true too much of the harmful kind of cholesterol in your bloodstream can increase your risk of clogged arteries, heart disease and stroke. And it's true that some foods are higher in cholesterol than others – prawns and eggs are notable examples.

But we now know that the cholesterol in our food isn't that important after all. Far more important is the cholesterol in our bloodstreams, and most of this is produced by our own bodies, by the liver.

So, instead of banning prawns, eggs and other foods demonised for containing dietary cholesterol, we should be cutting down on the foods that cause our livers to churn out too much of its own cholesterol.

And what are the main cholesterol-producing foods? Saturated fats – so that's yet another reason to cut down.

Not all fats are bad

Although we should all be making sure we don't eat too much fat (and especially not too much saturated and trans fats), it's wrong to be fat-phobic.

Certain kinds of fats – the unsaturated fats – are good for us in moderate quantities. We should make sure that most of the fats we eat are these healthy fats. For more on 'good fats', see chapter 2.

Sugar

Watch out for hidden sugars. As well as the sugar you put in your tea and coffee, you'll also find sugar in a variety of manufactured foods.

If you have a sweet tooth, you're not alone. The average intake of sugar in the UK is higher than it should be – and some people eat a lot more than the average. There's no denying it, sugar tastes good, and we're genetically programmed to be drawn to sweet tastes. And the body's natural fuel is glucose – the simplest kind of sugar. The problem is, humans aren't designed to eat large quantities of 'neat sugar' – they're designed to get their fuel from more complex forms of carbohydrate, which are gradually broken down to release a steady supply of sugar. In other words, our bodies prefer starchy foods such as bread and grains, especially the wholemeal versions.

Throughout history, sugar has been very hard to come by, and it's only comparatively recently that we've become surrounded by sweet treats. So now, our instincts tell us to shovel in the sugar, but our bodies wish we didn't! Too much sugar can lead to tooth decay and weight gain – and being overweight predisposes us to conditions such as heart disease, certain cancers, and type-2 diabetes. Sugar can also crowd out healthier foods from the diet – people grab a chocolate bar as a snack rather than an apple, or drink fizzy cola rather than water.

Sugary foods can also play havoc with our energy levels. Sugars are quickly absorbed by our bodies, leading to a rapid rise in our blood-sugar levels, and hence our energy levels. The problem is, this 'quick fix' is all too brief, and soon our blood sugar falls again, leaving us hungry, and often anxious and irritable. This makes us more likely to grab another chocolate muffin – it's a vicious circle.

We know that sugary foods aren't good for us, but how much is too much? The official recommendation is for us to get no more than 10 per cent of our calories from sugar. The recommended maximum daily sugar intake is:

- Average woman – 47g (approximately 9 teaspoons)
- Average man – 50g (approximately 10 teaspoons)

The main sources of sugar in the UK diet are:
- Fizzy drinks
- Sweets and chocolate
- Jams and other preserves

Some sugary manufactured foods are obvious, such as sweets, chocolates, fizzy drinks, biscuits, cakes and ice cream. And many sweetened foods such as fruit yogurts and other desserts are surprisingly high in sugar.

But you'll also find sugar 'hidden' in many foods that don't even taste sweet, including table sauces, chutneys and pickles, non-sweetened breakfast cereals (e.g. cornflakes and bran flakes), tinned spaghetti, tinned vegetables and baked beans, and even processed meat products (where sugar can be used to 'hold' water in the meat, in order to bulk it out).

So if you're trying to cut the amount of sugar in your diet, you'll need to read the labels for 'hidden' sugar, too.

Sugar appears on labels under a number of guises (you'll notice that many of them end in 'ose' – you can generally assume that any 'oses' on the label are sugars):

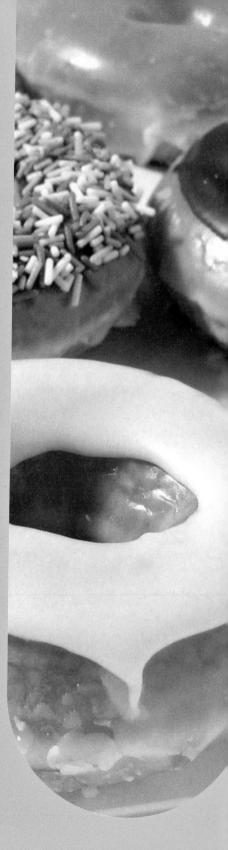

- Sucrose
- Glucose
- Dextrose
- Fructose
- Maltose
- High fructose corn syrup
- Corn syrup
- Corn sweetener
- Fruit juice concentrate
- Invert sugar
- Honey
- Molasses
- Raw sugar
- Syrup
- Malt syrup

New labelling regulations have tightened the rules on health claims concerning nutrients such as sugar – previously the rules were very 'woolly', with plenty of room for misinterpretation.

The new rules mean that:

- Reduced-sugar products must have at least 30 per cent less sugar than the 'standard' version
- Low-sugar products can't have more than 5g sugars per 100g for foods and no more than 2.5g of sugars per 100ml for drinks
- 'No added sugar' products are not allowed to contain added sugars, and if sugar is naturally found in that food, the label must say 'contains naturally occurring sugars'

However, although the new labelling rules are being phased in, companies have until 2009 before they are fully enforced.

> Avoid fizzy drinks – drink water or, if you need a sweeter taste, fresh fruit juice diluted with water instead.

Top tips

Cutting the sugar in your diet:

- Prepare your own food using unprocessed ingredients.
- Replace sweet snacks of chocolates, cakes or biscuits with fresh or dried fruit. Keep your fruit bowl full, and have a jar of sultanas and raisins, plus some unsalted nuts (almonds, Brazil nuts, hazelnuts and walnuts) handy. Then when you feel peckish, grab a small handful from the fruit jar and a couple of nuts from the nut jar for a sweet tasting snack that's high in nutrients and fibre. Try other dried fruit, such as apple, figs, prunes or unsulphured apricots, for a change.
- Look for the low-sugar options when buying sauces, baked beans and salad dressings (but beware of artificial sweeteners in 'sugar-free' varieties).
- When you're shopping at the supermarket, look for foods with a green 'traffic light label' for sugar.
- Base desserts around fresh fruit. Instead of a gooey dessert have a fresh fruit platter, with some natural yogurt or low-fat fromage frais for dipping.
- Instead of bought mousse or instant whips, stir mashed or puréed fruit into natural yogurt or low-fat fromage frais, for a delicious fruit fool. Mashed banana and puréed mango work particularly well. You can also sprinkle some chopped nuts or toasted seeds such as sesame seeds on top, for added crunch, plus a protein, fibre and omega-fatty acid boost.
- When you buy tinned fruit, buy it in its own juice or apple juice rather than in syrup.
- Bake your own cakes and biscuits – this means you can cut down the amount of sugar called for in the recipe. Many simple recipes, particularly if they contain natural sweeteners in the form of dried or mashed fruit, often don't need as much sugar as you'd think. Experiment, but be prepared for the occasional failure.
- Rather than using syrupy bought sauces, make fruit coulis to add to desserts. Simply whiz some mangoes, berries or other soft fresh fruit (use a mixture if you like) in a blender to make a sauce.
- Use non-sugar or low-sugar toppings for crackers, rice cakes and in sandwiches – reduced-sugar peanut butter, pure-fruit spreads and reduced-sugar jam, home-made hummus, low-fat cream cheese, or a yeast extract (use sparingly as it is high in salt). Watch out for sweeteners in peanut butter, spreads and jams.

- Avoid sugary breakfast cereals in favour of low-sugar, or no-added-sugar wholegrain cereals – check the labels to make sure. Sweeten them if you need to by adding some fresh or dried fruit, or a drizzle of honey.
- Make your own low-sugar muesli from oat flakes, nuts, seeds and dried fruit – that way there won't be any added sugar or salt, and you can base your recipe around your favourite ingredients.
- When you're feeling the need for something crunchy, don't grab a biscuit. Try a low-sugar snack, such as a few unsalted nuts, a handful of toasted sunflower or pumpkin seeds, or some plain popcorn.
- If you absolutely have to give in to your sweet tooth and only chocolate will do, have a square or two of good-quality chocolate (70 per cent cocoa solids or more, the darker the better) instead of a bar of chocolate candy.

'Good' sugars

When people talk about sugars and the health problems associated with them, they usually mean sucrose or 'table sugar', the kind that's generally added to cooking and to processed foods. But some sugars are healthier than others. Many fresh foods contain natural sugars. For example, fruit contains fructose, and milk contains lactose. But these sugars are less quickly absorbed by the body, sustaining us for longer. And in fruit and milk these natural sugars also come packaged with a whole variety of other nutrients – when you eat fruit you'll boost your intake of vitamins, minerals and fibre, and when you drink milk, you also get protein, calcium, and vitamins A and D.

What about pure fruit juice? It's high in vitamins, antioxidants and phyto-chemicals (beneficial plant chemicals), and you can count one 150ml glass of fruit juice towards your five-a-day fruit and vegetable target. But on the down-side fruit juice is also high in sugars (albeit natural ones) in a quick-release form – and it's acidic, so it can damage your teeth.

Always check the label when buying fruit juice – you're after 100 per cent pure with no added sugar or sweeteners.

Salt

Too much salt is bad for us, raising our blood pressure and increasing our risk of heart attacks and stroke. Too much salty food can also increase our risk of stomach cancer.

The official recommendation for maximum daily salt intake is 6g, but many of us eat too much. The average daily salt intake in the UK is 10.2g for men and 7.6 for women. That's slightly less than a few years ago – we are waking up to the fact that this is a serious matter – but we could do better!

The problem is, most of us are accustomed to salty tastes, and anything else can taste bland. But it is possible to retrain your taste buds in a surprisingly short time. Soon, you'll be experiencing the real taste of food – rather than the salt – and salty foods will taste unpleasant.

Where does salt come from? Obviously from the salt you add at the table, or during cooking. And some foods are obviously salty, such as anchovies, bacon, cheese, crisps and pretzels, olives, pickles, salted and dry roasted nuts, soy sauce, stock cubes and yeast extract (e.g. Marmite and Vegemite).

But, as with those other nutritional bugbears – saturated fat and sugar – much of the salt in our diets is 'hidden' – we need to track it down before we can avoid it. Many foods that don't taste particularly salty do in fact contain surprisingly high amounts of salt – and it all adds up. Watch out for the salt in sausages, smoked meat and fish, gravy granules and packet sauces, bread, crackers, breakfast cereals, biscuits (even sweet ones), tinned spaghetti, cook-in sauces, ready-meals, baked beans, table sauces such as tomato ketchup, tinned vegetables and beans, and soups.

Cutting the salt in your diet

When you're shopping:

- Around three-quarters of the salt we eat comes from processed foods, so the best thing you can do to reduce your salt intake is cut down on these, and cook as many of your meals as possible from scratch. That way you'll control the amount of salt that goes into what you eat.
- Read the labels – try to avoid foods with 1.25g salt or more per 100g (0.5g sodium or more per 100g) – this is a lot of salt.
- Aim for foods with 0.25g salt or less per 100g (0.1g sodium or less per 100g) – this is only a little salt (for a processed food).
- When you're shopping at the supermarket, look for foods with a green 'traffic light label' for salt.
- Cut down on foods from the obvious and not-so-obvious salty foods listed above.
- Buy nuts unsalted, rather than salted or packet dry-roasted (which have added salt and flavourings – home-roasted nuts are fine).

When you're cooking:

- Steam vegetables without salt, and then just add a very little during the last two minutes of cooking time.
- Look at the amount of salt you're adding while cooking. Don't just tip it into your hand and straight into the saucepan. Instead get a small spoon to use for salt and gradually decrease the amount you are adding over a few weeks. It's easier to see the amount you're using if you do this, and research has shown that if you cut down slowly no one will notice.
- If you're making a dish from a recipe, use half the amount of salt stated and only adjust the seasoning if necessary, just before it is ready to serve. You'll often find you don't need any more.
- Use herbs and spices to season your cooking, and make marinades and spicy rubs to add flavour to meat, poultry and fish, rather than seasoning with salt.
- Instead of buying ready-made pasta sauces, make your own using tinned tomatoes, and other vegetables such as onions, mushrooms, sweet peppers and sweetcorn, along with tomato juice, fresh herbs and ground black pepper. You can make it in the time it takes the pasta to cook.

If you buy pre-packed cheese, check the label for its salt content.

When you're eating:

- Watch how much cheese you eat. Cheese is a nutritious food, but it's generally high in fat and salt (blue and feta cheese are particularly salty). Eat cheese in small quantities, and go for strong-tasting cheeses (so you can get away with using less).
- Taste food before you add salt, and then only add a little at a time if you need it.
- Don't have salt on the dining table. If you have to go and get it, or your family has to ask for it, you might decide not to bother.

Reading the labels for salt

It's actually the sodium in salt that's bad for you, so many foods list sodium as well as or instead of salt – which can make things confusing.

Here's how to figure out how much salt you're getting:

- The amount of salt is the amount of sodium x 2.5
- So something that contains 1.5g of sodium per portion has 3.75g (i.e. 1.5g x 2.5) of salt per portion – which is well on the way towards your 6g maximum!

Remember to check that you know whether you're reading the amount per portion, or per 100g – it can make a huge difference.

Alcohol

Treated sensibly, there's nothing wrong with alcohol. A glass of wine with a meal, or the occasional drink socialising with friends, can enhance our lives. Alcohol in moderate amounts may even have health benefits for certain people (women after the menopause, and men over forty) by reducing our risk of heart attacks.

However, perhaps because alcohol plays such a large role in modern society, alcohol-related health problems are increasing.

Too much alcohol can lead to health problems including:

- Alcoholism
- Liver damage

- Weight gain and obesity
- Increased risk of liver, bowel, breast, oesophagus, mouth and larynx cancer
- Increased risk of type-2 diabetes
- Increased risk of heart disease, including heart-rhythm disturbances
- Stomach problems
- Sexual and fertility problems
- Risks to your baby, if you drink during pregnancy or the time of conception

Plus there are other less obvious problems – booze can also increase your risk of accidents, contribute to depression, interact dangerously with prescribed medication, disturb your sleep and deplete your body of nutrients (the B vitamins in particular). And we don't even have to mention the likelihood of a diabolical hangover the morning after if you overindulge!

How much is too much?

Moderation is the key. The maximum safe intake is:

- Women – 21 units of alcohol per week (2 to 3 units per day)
- Men – 28 units of alcohol per week (3 to 4 units per day).

You should also have at least a couple of alcohol-free days per week. And don't save your units for a weekend booze-up – binge drinking is especially dangerous.

Those units add up surprisingly quickly. Many people wrongly assume that an alcoholic drink equals a unit, simple as that. And in fact, in the past, it generally did.

But the problem is, the size of glass previously used to measure a unit of wine was a small glass, not the large glasses that many pubs and restaurants now serve as standard, which can raise your tally to one and a half or even two units per glass.

And don't forget that the measures of spirits you get at parties or serve at home tend to be more generous than pub measures, and an innocent-looking cocktail can hide four or five units in a single drink!

You also need to be aware of the alcoholic strength of your drinks. When units were devised, they were based on a 'standard strength' of wine, for example, which is 8 per cent alcohol by volume (abv). But nowadays we can buy wine up to 13 per cent abv. This means that a glass of wine served in a modern 'standard' glass can contain 2.3 units! Remember also that vintage cider contains more alcohol than ordinary cider, and premium lager contains more than standard lager.

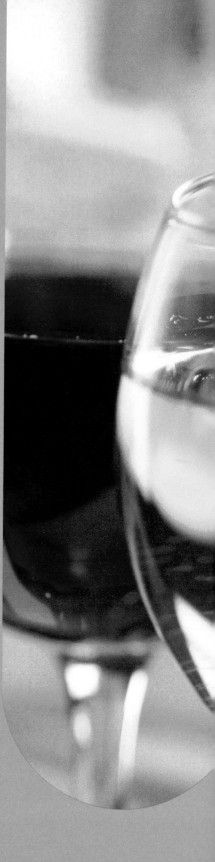

One unit is equal to:

- Half a pint of average-strength beer, lager or cider (3 to 4 per cent abv)
- A small glass of wine (8 per cent abv)
- A standard pub measure (25ml) of spirits (40 per cent abv)
- A standard pub measure (50 ml) of fortified wine, e.g. sherry or port (20 per cent abv)

And it's not just the alcohol in your drink that can harm your health. And booze can also pile on the pounds. Alcohol is surprisingly calorific, containing seven calories per gram (for comparison, fat contains nine per gram, and protein and carbohydrates both contain four calories per gram).

Sweet drinks also add to the calorie count, thanks to the calories in the added sugar – so watch out for sweet wines, liqueurs and alcopops. And mixers such as juice, cola, lemonade and the like can really make the sugar and calorie totals rise.

> Alcohol is surprisingly calorific so can have a big effect on your waistline as well as your health.

How many calories in your drink

Beers, lager and cider (per half-pint)

Bitter	90 calories
Mild bitter	71 calories
Pale ale	91 calories
Brown ale	80 calories
Lager – ordinary strength	85 calories
Low-alcohol lager	25 calories
Dry cider	95 calories
Sweet cider	110 calories

Wine (per small 125ml glass)

White wine (sweet)	118 calories
White wine (medium)	94 calories
White wine (dry)	83 calories

Sparkling white wine	95 calories
Red wine	85 calories
Rosé wine	89 calories

Fortified wine (per 50ml measure)
Port	79 calories
Sherry (dry)	58 calories

Spirits (per 25ml pub measure)
Gin, vodka, whisky, brandy, rum, etc.	52 calories

Liqueurs (per 25ml pub measure)
Cream liqueurs	81 calories
Tia Maria	66 calories
Grand Marnier	79 calories

Alcohol and pregnancy

If you drink during pregnancy, or when you are planning a baby, the alcohol could harm the developing baby or increase your risk of a miscarriage.

Previously, the advice was to limit your intake to a maximum of one or two units once or twice a week during this time. But, because some people appeared to be underestimating the risks, the government has recently strengthened its advice to women who are pregnant or planning to become pregnant, and now states that you should stop drinking entirely at this time.

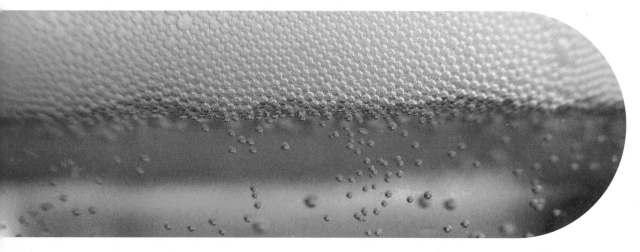

Processed and fast food

Because of our busy modern lives, it can be very tempting to rely on convenience and fast food, or to depend on them to make life easier.

Admittedly, there are times – for example when you're caught away from home and haven't had the chance to bring any healthy food with you, and if there isn't a healthy food outlet nearby – that you have to fall back on a less healthy alternative.

But processed and fast foods are often high in fat (especially saturated and trans fats), sugar, salt and artificial additives. So they certainly shouldn't be part of your everyday diet.

Processed food

Processing is generally done to make food more convenient for you (to make you more likely to buy it), or to increase its shelf life (making it more economical for the manufacturer). Unfortunately, nutrients are destroyed during the processing, and undesirable additives may be incorporated.

By making your meals and snacks from scratch, using fresh ingredients, you'll be maximising your intake of nutrients, and minimising your intake of chemicals that might be harmful. You'll also know exactly what goes into your food.

> Nutrients are destroyed during processing and undesirable additives may be incorporated

Convenient foods, not convenience foods

Not everything that comes in a tin or packet is bad for you! Take a look at the list below for some foods that make life easy for you, without compromising your nutritious diet:

- Tinned tomatoes
- Tinned fruit in juice
- Tinned fish (salmon, pilchards, sardines, mackerel, tuna)
- Tinned sweetcorn (choose no-salt, no-sugar)
- Tinned beans (such as kidney beans and chickpeas) and lentils – these are often canned in salty brine, so rinse before use
- UHT milk
- Some breakfast cereals (such as no-sugar, no-salt muesli, wholewheat bisks) – wholegrain low-sugar, no-salt cereals that are fortified with vitamins and minerals are good for children

Fast food

Fast food is everywhere, from burgers, crispy-crumbed chicken and fries, to pizza, kebabs, Indian and Chinese takeaways.

The problem is, much of this food is deep-fried, and hence loaded with fat. And many fast-food chains still fry in hydrogenated (trans) fats.

Drinks at fast-food chains can be nutritionally dire – thick milk shakes are full of fat, sugar and calories, and fizzy drinks are basically a tooth-rotting solution of chemicals sweetened with either sugar or artificial sweeteners (even diet drinks are acidic, so can harm your teeth).

Fast food is also notoriously low in fruit and vegetables, fibre, vitamins and minerals. If you eat fast food, not only are you loading up your body with unhealthy anti-nutrients, you're also missing out on the nutrients your body desperately needs.

For all these reasons, fast food and unhealthy processed food shouldn't be part of your healthy-eating plan. If you must occasionally fall back on these less healthy choices, read the labels (in fast-food chains, see if they have a nutritional leaflet) and carry out some 'damage limitation':

- **Go for the lowest fat content possible:** The Food Standards Agency (FSA) says that 20g fat per 100g food is 'a lot of fat', and 5g saturated fat per 100g food is 'a lot of saturated fat'. Reduced-fat foods have to contain at least 30 per cent less fat than the 'standard' version, but this may still be extremely high in fat, making the concept of 'reduced' rather dubious. Foods labelled 'low-fat' contain no more than 3g fat per 100g.

- **Watch out for high sugar:** The FSA guidelines say that 10g sugars or more per 100g food is 'a lot', and 2g sugars per 100g food is 'a little'. If a label says a food is 'low-sugar', it contains no more than 5g sugars per 100g. A low-sugar drink can't contain more than 2.5g sugars per 100ml. Reduced-sugar foods and drinks contain at least 30 per cent less sugar than the 'standard' version, but this could still be extremely sugary, so 'reduced' might still be high in sugar.

- **Go for low salt:** The FSA guidelines say that 1.25g salt (0.5g sodium) per 100g food is 'a lot', and 0.25g salt (0.1g sodium) per 100g food is 'a little'. Foods labelled 'low-sodium' or 'low-salt' contain no more than 0.12g sodium per 100g or 100ml, which is equivalent to no more than 0.3g salt per 100g or 100ml.

- Also, avoid hydrogenated (trans) fats wherever possible.

Get into the habit of checking the labels on the food you buy for their fat, sugar and salt content.

Additives

Additives are added to foods for a variety of reasons:

- To make food look and taste better
- To prevent food from spoiling and keep it safe for consumption
- To make food cheaper and easier to manufacture
- To make it 'healthier' (for example by artificially boosting its vitamin content)

Food additives are nothing new. We've been salting and smoking food, pickling it and making it into jams and preserves for centuries, if not millennia. But the range of additives available to modern food scientists is a far cry from the limited list of history, and many of them are only there for the manufacturer's benefit. They can make food less nutritious, and some may even be harmful when eaten in large quantities.

It's impossible to avoid additives totally. Without preservatives, for example, we would be at high risk of serious food poisoning. However, it makes sense to minimise your intake of unnecessary additives.

Preservatives

Preservatives include ingredients such as salt (for example in bacon) and sugar (as in jams) – they stop the food from growing mouldy and increase its keeping properties. Although we need to reduce the salt and sugar in our diets, when we talk about preservatives in the context of food additives, we generally mean the artificial chemicals added by the food industry. These include sodium benzoate (E211), sulphur dioxide (E220) and potassium sorbate (E202).

Flavourings and flavour enhancers

Good, tasty and healthy food doesn't need artificial flavourings or flavour enhancers. The food industry adds these to mask poor-quality ingredients, and to make up for the fact that many processed foods are low in the healthy ingredients that would give them taste. For example, a 'strawberry flavour' yogurt that doesn't contain any real strawberries will need artificial flavourings to give it a fruity taste.

There's also a loophole that means the over 4,500 artificial flavourings available to food manufacturers don't have to be listed by name on the label. All you will see is the word 'flavourings', no matter how many or what they are.

Flavour enhancers are added to foods to increase the strength of the taste they do have. The most familiar is monosodium glutamate, also known as MSG or E621. Monosodium glutamate brings out the savoury taste of food. It's commonly added to food at Chinese restaurants and takeaways. Most people can eat MSG without problems (it occurs naturally in foods such as Parmesan cheese and mushrooms), but if you are sensitive to it you may experience symptoms such as headaches.

Artificial sweeteners

Artificial sweeteners are used to replace sugar in food for two reasons. They're added to 'diet' foods and 'diabetic' foods, because they're much lower in calories than sugar, and don't cause a rise in blood sugar in the way that 'real' sugar does. However, 'diet' and 'diabetic' foods are generally a potentially unhealthy waste of money. People wanting to lose weight, and diabetics, would be far better eating real food, and simply watching their sugar intake, relying on natural sugars from fruit, and only the smallest amount of refined sugar. (Diabetics should always follow the dietary advice of their dietician and diabetic nurse.)

Artificial sweeteners are also added to foods because, perhaps surprisingly, they are cheaper than 'real' sugar. For this reason you'll also find them on the ingredients lists of many non-diet foods, such as tinned spaghetti and baked beans, sauces, dressings, pickles, and baked goods such as biscuits and bars.

Although there is no actual scientific proof that artificial sweeteners are dangerous, some studies suggest that they may be bad for us, particularly when we consume a lot of them (perhaps you know someone who drinks litres of 'diet' fizz?).

And although all the additives in our food have been passed as 'safe', there is some concern that, because we eat so many different foods that are laced with chemicals, the huge range of additives could form a kind of 'chemical cocktail' inside our bodies, with effects that we don't yet understand.

Also, artificial sweeteners do nothing to dull our 'sweet tooth', which is what we want in the long run, so that we will naturally prefer the healthier wholefoods. If you're accustomed to intensely sweet foods, a healthy food like an orange, for example, whose sweetness comes from natural sugars, may taste 'sour'. You just need to blunt your sweet tooth, so that you naturally prefer healthy sweet foods, such as fruit – both fresh and dried.

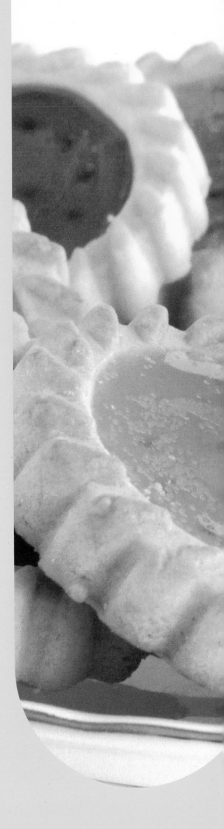

Know your sweeteners

Probably the best-known artificial sweetener is aspartame. You may also see it on the label as E951, Nutrasweet™, Equal™, Canderel™, Spoonful™, Benevia™ or 'contains a source of phenylalanine'.

Other artificial sweeteners include saccharin (E954 or Sweet 'N' Low, commonly used as a tabletop sweetener), acesulfame K (E950), sucralose (E955, or Splenda), and xylitol (E967).

Artificial colourings

Colourings are added to make food look more attractive. For example, when some foods are processed, they turn an unappetising sludgy grey or brown, so colourings are added to make them look the way we think they should. And foods that are low in 'real' ingredients may also have added colourings, as in the case of some fruit desserts and yogurts. A raspberry yogurt or dessert made with real fruit and other wholesome ingredients will naturally be a pale pink colour – but some brands are a lurid magenta! Do we really need food to be that colour? Unfortunately, many foods aimed at children are highly coloured. Kids love bright colours, and chemicals are added to make foods appeal to them. Fortunately, many manufacturers are removing artificial colourings from their foods (especially those targeted at children) – so check the label, or look for a 'no artificial colourings' flash on the packaging. Or – best of all – avoid the processed foods entirely and make your own from fresh ingredients. A low-fat natural yogurt with some mango purée swirled in is delicious, and far better for you than a bought yogurt with added sugar, sweeteners, flavourings and colourings.

Caffeine

Some people are sensitive to the stimulant effects of caffeine, and it can cause symptoms of shakiness, jitteriness and anxiety. Caffeine can also keep you awake, and its effect is likely to be particularly strong if you're caffeine-sensitive.

It's a good idea to avoid coffee (generally the main source of caffeine in our diets) after lunchtime, in order to get a good night's sleep. And if you're caffeine-sensitive, it's probably a good idea to watch your intake of other caffeinated foods and drinks after lunch, too.

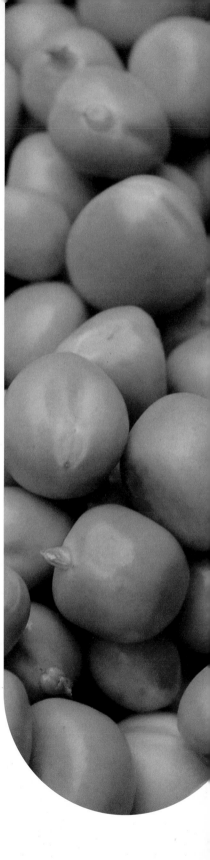

Sources of caffeine:

- Shot of espresso – 130mg
- Cup of brewed coffee – 90mg caffeine
- Cup of instant coffee – 60mg
- Cup of tea – 40mg
- Can of cola – up to 70mg
- Can of energy drink – up to 70mg
- 50g chocolate bar – 10mg
- Cup of hot chocolate – 5mg
- Some painkillers and cold remedies – check the label.

Despite their popularity, nutritionally speaking there's nothing going for cola drinks, and a lot to say against them. Do without them! Energy drinks are no better – just sweetened water with additives. Sports drinks are slightly different – these are specially formulated to aid hydration. But even though they have a purpose, they're of no benefit unless you're a serious athlete.

The advantages of organic food

As well as the artificial preservatives, colourings, sweeteners and flavourings that are added as 'ingredients' to our food, we also need to be aware of pesticide residues that can remain on food crops, such as fruit, vegetables and cereal grains (such as those used to make flour).

Food products are checked at random to ensure that their pesticide residue levels are below the levels deemed safe. And – apart from the occasional story you read about in the news – the food we eat does remain in the 'safe zone'.

But is it a good idea to be eating any of these chemicals?

Eating organic is probably the best thing you can do to minimise your intake of potentially harmful pesticides, animal medications and some chemical food additives. On packaged food, look for the Soil Association's logo.

What's different about organic food?

- Under organic standards, only four out of the hundreds of available pesticides may be used on crops, and this only as a last resort.
- It minimises the use of additives.

- It isn't allowed to contain genetically modified (GM) ingredients.
- Conventional farmers sometimes use veterinary medicines on animals as a preventative measure, which can lead to residues of the drugs ending up in our meat and poultry. Organic farmers only use medicines on animals that are actually ill, minimising the chance of these chemicals ending up in our food.
- Some organic foods appear to be higher in nutrients. For example, organic chicken contains lower levels of fat than non-organic chicken, and organic milk contains higher levels of omega-3 essential fatty acids, vitamin E and the antioxidant betacarotene.

And many people say organic food simply tastes better. This seems perfectly reasonable – without the artificial 'help' provided by drugs and chemicals, food is allowed to grow and ripen, and animals allowed to mature, slowly and naturally. This will, for example, lead to more tasty natural sugars in slow-ripened tomatoes.

Things that aren't allowed in organic food:

- GM (genetically modified)
- Hydrogenated (trans) fats
- Aspartame (an artificial sweetener)
- Monosodium glutamate (MSG – a flavour enhancer)
- Phosphoric acid (a chemical that can damage teeth and increase the risk of bone thinning; found in cola drinks)
- Sulphur dioxide (an artificial preservative)

Remember, however, that 'organic' doesn't necessarily mean healthy. You can still buy organic biscuits, cakes and ready-meals for example. They won't contain the chemicals we've already mentioned, but they can still be high in fat, sugar and salt. It's just organically produced fat, sugar and salt!

Top tips
Minimising the additives:

- Cook it yourself – using additive-free wholefoods such as fruit and vegetables, lean meat, poultry and fish, eggs, dairy products and wholegrains. In other words, foods without ingredients lists.
- Buy organic – to minimise your intake of both additives and pesticide residues.

- Grow it yourself – this way you can get organic produce at a fraction of the cost. And it will be so much fresher than fruit and vegetables from the supermarket.

What to buy organic

Organic food is undeniably more expensive than non-organic. But it's worth buying organic whenever you can afford it. Make these your priorities:

- Meat and poultry
- Salmon
- Vegetables that won't be peeled, especially lettuce
- Carrots (a lot of chemicals are used on conventionally farmed carrots)
- Fruits where the skin is eaten, such as apples and grapes
- Tea and coffee (if you don't buy organic, these are generally intensively sprayed with chemicals)

Bad Eating Habits

If we're honest, most of us have some bad eating habits. Perhaps you skip breakfast, or miss lunch when you're busy. Or maybe you eat on the hoof, rather than sitting down. Perhaps your family never sits down to eat a proper meal together. If you count buying fast food as a 'habit', you could add that to the list, too!

Skipping meals

Skipping meals can make it harder for our bodies to maintain steady blood-sugar levels, and hence can lead to dips in energy levels. Eating regular meals and healthy snacks, on the other hand, particularly when they're based around 'slow-release' fuel in the form of wholegrain carbohydrates, fruit and vegetables, with low-fat protein, is much healthier. This kind of eating pattern produces a steady drip-feed of fuel for our bodies, rather than a sudden 'spike' followed just as rapidly by a fall.

Also, if you skip meals, you're less likely to hit your vitamin and mineral targets for the day. If you miss breakfast or lunch so that you're extra-hungry later on, you're very likely to make up for the missed calories when you next eat. But when you're ravenous, your food choices are likely to be less healthy. Skipping breakfast before you leave home, for example, makes you more likely to grab a Danish pastry on the way to work, or to raid the biscuit barrel once you get there.

Breakfast is the meal most people are likely to miss, but skipping it is a really bad habit.

Don't rush your food. Guzzling down a meal makes you more likely to over eat

Skipping breakfast is a particularly bad habit, and unfortunately, breakfast is the meal people are most likely to miss, particularly if they are trying to lose weight, or in a hurry in the morning.

Eating too fast

Don't guzzle your food – if you wolf it down as though it's going to be taken away from you, you're more likely to overeat. As your stomach fills up with food and expands, and slightly later as the products of digestion are absorbed, your body sends 'stop eating' messages to your brain. If you gobble your food, by the time you receive the message, you'll already have eaten too much!

Gobbling – particularly if you're talking at the same time – makes it more likely that you'll swallow air, leading to uncomfortable bloating and wind.

You also shouldn't drink large amounts while you're eating, to avoid diluting the digestive juices in your stomach. Sips of water with your meal are fine, though sparkling water can make you feel bloated, especially when drunk with food. And fizzy sweetened drinks shouldn't even be part of your healthy diet.

Eating on the run

With today's fast-paced lifestyles, we're often forced to grab a meal 'on the hoof'. But this isn't a habit you should get into, for several reasons:

- You have less control over the food you eat
- If you fall into the fast-food trap, you'll probably be eating too much fat, salt and probably sugar
- You're more likely to overeat, since you won't be concentrating fully on your food
- If you don't allow time to chew your food well and give your body time to digest it properly, you'll increase the likelihood of suffering from indigestion, or a growling gut and wind thanks to swallowed air!
- It's more expensive

Not eating together

It's a sad reflection on modern life that so few families eat together these days. Adult family members get home from work at different times, and often very late. Children have various out-of-school activities to attend, and homework to do. And everyone wants to have a social life!

So, the traditional sit-down family meal is being abandoned in favour of individual microwave meals, fast food grabbed on the way to work, and pub suppers washed down with plenty of alcohol.

Try to eat as many of your meals together as you can. It doesn't always have to be the evening meal – that might not always be practical. How about trying always to eat together at the weekends, and making Sunday breakfasts 'special'?

Eating together is an ideal time for the family to 'bond', and for people to get anything that's bothering them off their chest. This makes it perfect for discussing new foods you'd like to try. Mealtimes are also opportunities to persuade children to eat more healthily. For a start, they're more likely to choose healthy food if you show that you enjoy it too. And when you introduce something new to the family's meals, you can explain what it is, and provide encouragement for young fussy eaters.

Research has shown that families that eat together, eat healthier. Frequent family meals are linked to a higher intake of nutrients (for everyone), children doing better at school, and less risk of unhealthy dieting and eating disorders among teenagers. Children of families who eat together regularly were also found to be happier with life in general.

Fad Diets

More than 25 per cent of the population says that they are on a weight-loss diet for 'most of the time', and on top of that there's a huge number of people who are 'on and off' diets.

Sadly, far too many people embark on crash diets, or trendy diets endorsed by celebrities but with little (if any) scientific proof behind them. People want a quick fix – we want to be slim and gorgeous NOW, so we fall for fad diets that promise the world.

The 'bad' diets – we'll call them Fad Diets – are neither safe nor effective. They may enable you to lose weight (and often quite a lot of weight) quickly. But because they generally ignore the rules of good nutrition in favour of a quick fix, they can be dangerous.

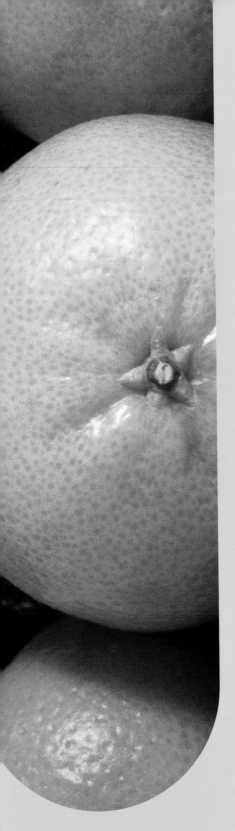

And in the long run, Fad Diets aren't even effective. Although the weight comes off initially, these diets don't address the root cause of the problem – not eating a healthy balanced diet in the first place – so people eventually slip back into their old ways. And the weight creeps or piles back on. Eventually, most dieters choosing Fad Diets end up fatter than before.

This leads to a sad cycle of 'yo-yo' dieting, where people lurch between rapid weight loss, and putting it back on again. Not only is this horribly discouraging, it's also bad for your health.

Problems with Fad Diets

- When you greatly reduce your food intake, you reduce your intake of valuable nutrients. Your body needs a certain amount of protein, fat and carbohydrates, not to mention vitamins and minerals, in order to thrive. (The You Are What You Eat way of eating recommends eating plenty of healthy food.)
- Drastically reducing your calorie intake will leave you hungry, weak and miserable. Being constantly hungry is no fun.
- You need good, sustaining food to give you the energy for the exercise that's essential for sustained weight loss and good health.
- Fad Diets often soon become boring, particularly if they revolve around one or more 'magic' ingredients such as cabbage, celery or grapefruit.
- Cutting out food groups (such as wheat and dairy) can lead to nutrient deficiencies and imbalances, even if you try to make up the shortfall with supplements.
- Strange, faddy eating patterns can lead to an unhealthy obsession with food, which could progress into an eating disorder.

How to sniff out a Fad Diet

Avoid any diet that:

- Promises miracles. If it sounds too good to be true, it is!
- Cuts out entire food groups, such as wheat or dairy. Although some people are genuinely allergic or intolerant to certain foods, this is neither a safe nor sensible method of weight loss.
- Concentrates on one kind of food, such as celery, cabbage or raw food.
- Involves taking pills or supplements to boost your metabolism or quell your hunger. You can do these things, but by exercising and eating the right foods, not by popping a pill.

- Involves fasting. Your body needs a steady supply of food and nutrients. Fasting – especially for some people with medical conditions – can be dangerous.
- Focuses only on your looks (i.e. 'get thin at all costs') rather than on all-round good health and vitality.

Diet and exercise

If you want to lose weight, you need to look at both your diet and exercise. Research has shown that dieting is the most popular way of losing weight, but cutting calories without initiating a sensible exercise programme can lead to loss of bone density, increasing your risk of osteoporosis.

The dangers of being underweight

While the dangers of carrying too much weight are generally well known, fewer people realise that being underweight can also lead to health problems.

Sadly, a worrying number of people seem to have an unhealthy fixation with the kind of figures possessed by catwalk models, and dream of slimming down to the unrealistic 'size zero' (a UK size 4) idealised in some fashion magazines.

For almost everyone on the planet, this kind of figure is simply neither practical nor safe. To get (and stay) that thin, you would have to virtually starve yourself, making yourself miserable in the process. The misery wouldn't just be caused by being deprived of good food, but also because of the nutrient imbalances you'd set up in your body and brain. And that's before you consider the harm that being such a low weight poses to your health.

Being underweight can lead to many problems:

- It can lead to women having irregular periods or their periods stopping completely
- This can cause bone thinning, increasing the risk of osteoporosis
- The hormone changes caused by being underweight can lead to fertility problems

- Being underweight can encourage an unhealthy attitude towards food and your diet, increasing the risk of eating disorders
- If you don't have enough insulation in the form of body fat, you can suffer badly from the cold, and even minor bumps and bruises will be very painful
- If an actual eating disorder does develop, such as anorexia nervosa or bulimia, this can lead to serious health problems in the long run, and even death
- Even if a 'full-blown' eating disorder doesn't develop, the kind of 'disordered eating' shown by many people who have or are trying to slim down to an unrealistic so-called 'ideal', can lead to nutrient deficiencies that harm their long-term health and, in the short term, make them feel below par

The most important thing is to be the right weight for YOU. This means maintaining a healthy weight, with a diet providing all the nutrients you need, and an exercise routine that gives your body the physical activity it requires to stay strong and fit. It's healthier to be slightly chunky in build, but with the right balance of muscle to body fat, than to be scrawny, anxious and at risk from several potentially serious health problems.

Top tips

- Eat regular meals and healthy snacks
- Don't skip meals – breakfast is especially important
- Don't gobble your food
- Try not to eat 'on the run' – make time for a break
- Have at least one sit-down family meal every day
- Beware Fad Diets – make sure you eat enough healthy food

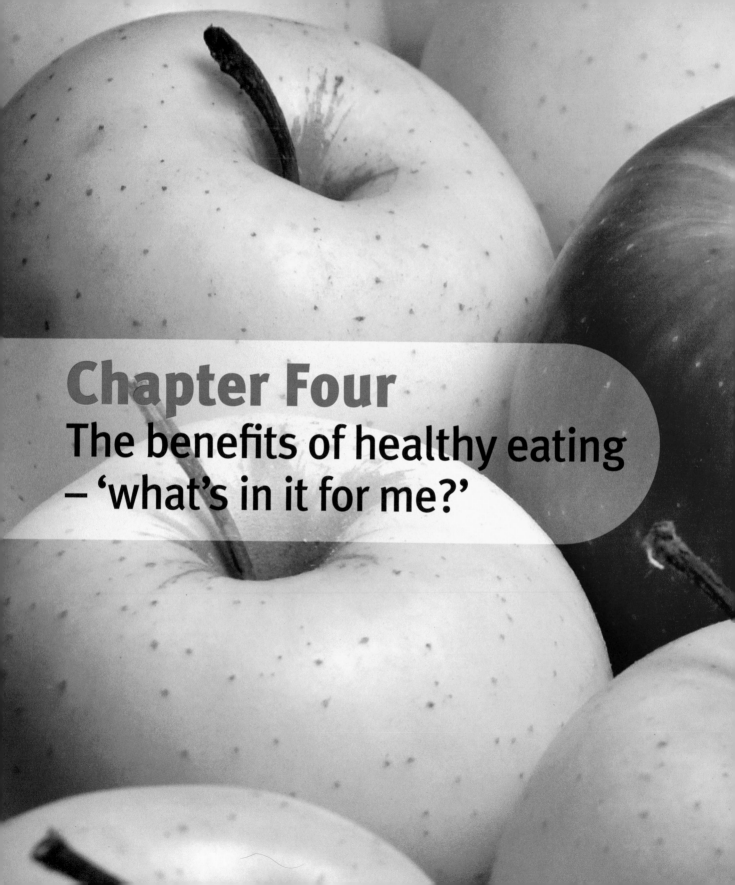

Chapter Four
The benefits of healthy eating – 'what's in it for me?'

you are™
what
you eat

Healthy eating – what's the big deal?

Fortunately, most of the serious nutritional deficiencies, like scurvy (a serious vitamin C deficiency), have been eradicated in this country. But there's still a significant number of people with 'sub-clinical' deficiencies – not serious enough to register as an actual deficiency, but their intakes are still not quite high enough, so they may feel below par, run down or tired. Also, if you're poorly nourished, your risk of illness – both everyday minor sniffles, and also the big killer diseases we all fear – increases.

To spell it out bluntly, most of us would feel a whole lot better, and probably live longer, if we ate better!

Short-term Benefits

More energy

Do you feel tired all the time, listless and lethargic? Your diet could be at least partly to blame.

Perhaps you've got a bit of a junk-food habit, or you rely on fast food to save time. Beware! The mainstays of your diet will be high in calories, fat and sugar, and although they may taste good, they don't keep you full for long, and the energy they supply is soon gone. Far better to fill up with tasty wholefoods that will keep you going for ages.

Great foods for energy

Oats: full of soluble fibre, which is also good for your heart and circulatory system, as well as your digestive system.

Bananas: rich in starch, and also a great source of heart-healthy potassium.

Nuts: Provide energy in the form of healthy unsaturated fats. Also good for vitamin E and protein.

Brown rice: provides slow-release starchy carbohydrate, as well as a good source of the B vitamins.

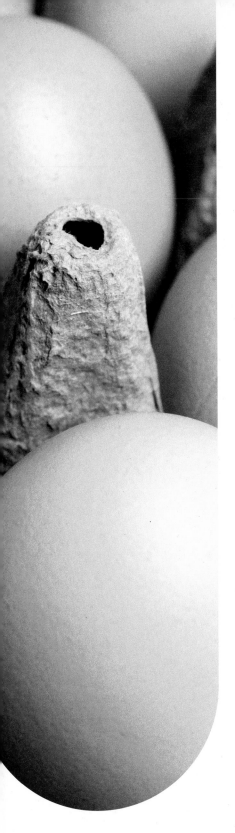

More stable moods

If you're eating a poor diet, particularly if you eat too much sugar, your blood-sugar levels may well be all over the place.

The body has its own very good systems to keep blood sugar within safe limits, so it won't let them rise or fall to dangerous levels. When your blood-sugar level rises, your pancreas produces insulin, which squirrels the sugar away and brings your blood sugar back to normal. The exception is in people with diabetes – their body is either unable to produce enough insulin, or to respond to the insulin it does produce, so blood sugar can rise and plummet to dangerous levels.

However, although most of us are able to keep our blood sugar at safe levels, some people seem to be particularly sensitive to its rises and falls. The result? They feel buzzy and low by turns, and may suffer mood swings.

If you always reach for a sugary snack when you're hungry, you can get into a cycle of quickly getting hungry again, knowing that you oughtn't stave off the hunger with some chocolate or biscuits, feeling anxious and crabby – and then eating them anyhow. Which keeps the whole vicious circle going. It's far better to stop the cycle in its tracks with a healthy, sustaining snack such as a couple of oatcakes spread with low-fat soft cheese, or a small handful of raisins and unsalted nuts. These will properly quell your hunger, and keep you going until your next meal.

Also, people who are deficient in certain nutrients are more likely to suffer from depression. So, it seems reasonable that eating a good, balanced diet will not only make us less likely to get depressed, but also help us to keep our emotions on an even keel.

Good mood foods

Eating the 'energy foods' on page 90 will help to keep your blood-sugar levels stable, in case you're sensitive to even minor wobbles in blood sugar. Low levels of certain vitamins and minerals are associated with an increased risk of depression. So it stands to reason that we should try to eat plenty of foods containing as much as possible of these nutrients, if we want to stay happy:

- Oily fish (such as salmon and mackerel): rich in omega-3 essential fatty acids, which are linked with a decreased risk of depression
- Brazil nuts: rich in the mineral selenium

- Lean meat and low-fat dairy products: high in the mineral magnesium
- Wholegrains, such as brown rice, wholemeal bread and brown pasta: sources of magnesium that are suitable for vegetarians
- Eggs: high in folate, one of the B vitamins
- Green leafy vegetables: also great for folate

Less PMS

A lot of the symptoms of pre-menstrual syndrome are linked with diet. A lack of certain vitamins, minerals and essential fatty acids can make your symptoms worse, and so can eating too much of certain foods.

Caffeine, and too much salt, can make the symptoms of PMS worse. Cut them out (or cut them down drastically) in the fortnight before your period is due. If you suffer particularly badly from PMS, try totally removing them from your diet (or cutting down on them as much as possible).

PMS-beating foods

Wholegrains

Foods like wholemeal bread, brown rice and brown pasta help to relieve mood swings and keep your energy levels stable.

Oily fish

Salmon, mackerel, sardines, trout, pilchards and fresh tuna are all good sources of omega-3 essential fatty acids, which appear to relieve some of the physical and mood-based symptoms of PMS.

Evening primrose oil:

The oil from the evening primrose plant can relieve the symptoms of some women who suffer from painful breasts before their period. You can buy evening primrose oil in capsule or liquid form – ask your doctor or a registered nutritionist or dietician for advice on dosage, and whether it's suitable for you.

Better skin and hair

If you're eating badly, it's likely to show in the condition of your skin and hair.

Great foods for skin and hair

These are the main nutrients you need to keep your skin clear and glowing, and your hair smooth and lustrous.

Vitamin A

A deficiency can lead to rough, dry skin. You can find this vitamin in meat (especially liver), eggs and dairy products, as well as green, orange and yellow fruit and vegetables.

Essential fatty acids

Healthy unsaturated fats are needed to maintain the natural oils in our skin. You can find these 'good fats' in nuts and seeds, oils such as olive, sunflower and sesame oil, and also oily fish.

Vitamin C

This is needed for the production of collagen, a protein that helps to keep the skin stretchy and resilient, and helps to prevent premature wrinkles. Get your vitamin C from rich sources such as blackcurrants, oranges and other citrus fruits, kiwi fruits and strawberries.

Water

Dehydration can make your skin dry and flaky.

Lose weight – if you need to

You don't need to be a genius to realise that eating a bad diet can make you pile on the pounds. If you follow the advice in this book, you'll shed any excess pounds – slowly, safely, sustainably – without feeling deprived.

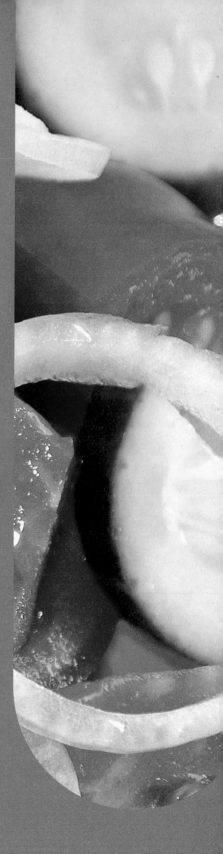

Top foods for safe weight loss

- **Wholegrains:** For sustained energy, to help you resist unhealthy snacks.
- **Big salads:** To fill you up, and help you on your way to your five-a-day target for fruit and vegetables.
- **Fruit snacks:** Have an apple, orange or banana, rather than a bar of chocolate or packet of crisps.
- **Fish:** White fish (such as haddock, cod and plaice) are great sources of protein, and extremely low in fat and calories. Oily fish (salmon, tuna, etc.) is higher in fat, but has extra health benefits for your heart and blood vessels. Other good low-fat protein sources are chicken and turkey.
- **Water:** Many people think they're hungry when in fact they're just thirsty. Keep hydrated!

Long-term Benefits

As well as making you feel better right now, and helping you to live life to the full, eating a healthy diet can also reduce your risk of suffering the serious chronic diseases that spoil your quality of life, and even cut your life short.

Eating nutritious food can:

- Keep your arteries healthy and fur-free
- Reduce your risk of heart disease and stroke
- Lower your blood pressure
- Reduce your risk of certain cancers, especially breast, bowel, uterus and stomach cancers
- Reduce your risk of type-2 diabetes
- Reduce your risk of arthritis
- Give you more energy for exercise and enjoying life
- Help you to stay active as you grow older, so you're more likely to enjoy a healthy old age

Eating for healthy blood vessels

Eating a heart-healthy diet reduces the risk of damage and clogging to your arteries. 'Furred up' arteries are likely to produce life-threatening clots, or to become blocked, causing a heart attack (if the blockage is in the heart), a stroke (if it occurs in the brain), or deep vein thrombosis (if the blockage occurs in one of the major veins, such as in the legs).

Maintaining a healthy weight, and eating the right foods, helps to keep your arteries smooth and healthy.

Top foods for smooth arteries:

- Eat plenty of fruit and vegetables, and nuts and seeds. Their antioxidants protect your artery walls from damage.
- Eat healthy unsaturated fats, such as olive oil, rather than saturated and trans fats.
- Eat oily fish at least twice a week (but no more than twice if you're pregnant or planning a baby).
- Eat garlic – it can help lower your levels of 'bad' LDL cholesterol.
- Have your blood pressure and cholesterol levels checked regularly.

Artery enemies:

- Too much fat in your diet – it can lead to obesity
- Too much alcohol (limit yourself to a maximum of a drink or two in a day)
- Saturated and trans (hydrogenated) fats – these increase your levels of the harmful kind of cholesterol that contributes to damaged and blocked arteries

Eating to lower your blood pressure

High blood pressure increases your risk of heart attack and stroke, but you can help keep it low by eating a diet that's low in sodium and salt. Potassium-rich foods are also good for maintaining a healthy blood pressure – so eat more nuts (especially almonds and hazelnuts), and sprinkle sesame seeds on your cereal and salads, use them in baking, and add to stir-fries. Bananas are a great potassium-rich snack, and lentils and green leafy vegetables are good for this mineral, too.

Eating to prevent cancer

If you want to protect yourself from cancer, the best two things you can do is stop smoking (or don't start in the first place) and eat a healthy diet – up to 40 per cent of cancers are caused by a poor diet. Maintaining a healthy weight is important too as is exercise.

Top anti-cancer foods:

- Eat plenty of fruit and vegetables – they're rich in immune-boosting nutrients, and a strong immune system can protect you from cancer, as well as other diseases.
- Concentrate on fruits that are packed with antioxidants, such as blueberries, prunes, raisins and strawberries.
- Eat plenty of fibre, found in fruit, vegetables, wholegrains and pulses, to help maintain a healthy weight (being obese increases your cancer risk). Also, fibre speeds the passage of waste products through the bowel, limiting the amount of time potential carcinogens (cancer-causing chemicals) spend in contact with the bowel wall, and this helps protect you from bowel cancer.
- Eat lots of cabbage, broccoli, cauliflower and Brussels sprouts. They contain phytochemicals (plant chemicals) called isothiocyanates, which are thought to help protect against cancer.
- Eat nuts and seeds – they're rich in vitamin E and selenium, both powerful antioxidants.

> Eating plenty of fruit and vegetables can help protect against diseases including cancer

Foods to avoid:

- Don't eat too much processed and red meat – a high intake of these kinds of meat are linked with an increased bowel cancer risk. A couple of times a week is fine.
- Don't drink too much alcohol – stay within the safe limit of two to three units a day for women, and three to four units for men, with at least two or three alcohol-free days a week.
- Reduce your salt intake – high-salt diets increase your stomach cancer risk.
- Don't eat charred or burned food – it can contain carcinogens.

Healthy eating vs type-2 diabetes

People who suffer from diabetes cannot regulate their blood-sugar levels effectively. There are two main kinds of diabetes – types 1 and 2. Type-1 diabetes usually begins in children or young people, but type-2 diabetes generally shows symptoms at a later age – that's why it used to be called 'adult-onset diabetes'. However, a lot of the risk of developing this condition is down to diet and lifestyle, and thanks to today's junk-food and couch-potato habits, it's being seen in younger people, and even children.

Thankfully, there's a lot you can do to reduce your risk.

How to reduce your type-2 diabetes risk:

- Maintain a healthy weight – this is particularly important if you are an 'apple shape' who stores their body fat around their middle. Obese women are almost thirteen times more likely to develop type-2 diabetes than non-obese women, while obese men are nearly five times more likely to develop the illness.
- Reduce your total fat intake, and eat moderate amounts of 'good' mono- and polyunsaturated fats.
- Reduce the amount of processed and fast food you eat.

The typical candidate for type-2 diabetes is an overweight woman (though men aren't exempt!) who stores fat around her middle rather than her bottom and thighs, eats an unhealthy diet and doesn't exercise enough. Make sure this isn't you!

Eating to prevent arthritis
There's a lot you can do to keep your joints smooth and pain-free into old age.

Top tips
- Maintain a healthy weight – carrying too many pounds means extra wear and tear on your joints.
- Eat oily fish, sprinkle flaxseeds on your cereal, and consider taking an omega-3 supplement. Omega-3 essential fatty acids are involved in maintaining healthy joints, and getting plenty of omega-3s can delay or prevent the development of osteoarthritis.

Eating to prevent osteoporosis
Eating for strong, healthy bones (especially in the years up to your early thirties, when you reach your peak bone density) reduces your risk of osteoporosis later in life. Aim to eat foods high in calcium, which makes up much of the solid structure of bone.

Top anti-osteoporosis foods:
- Tofu
- Low-fat dairy products
- Tinned fish where the bones are eaten
- Beans such as red kidney beans, baked beans and chickpeas
- Sesame seeds
- Dried figs

You also need vitamin D, to enable the calcium to be absorbed and used. Your body makes its own vitamin D from the effect of sunlight on the skin, but you can also find vitamin D in foods such as oily fish, meat, eggs, dairy products and fortified breakfast cereals and spreads.

Eating to prevent Alzheimer's

Certain foods seem to reduce the risk of Alzheimer's and other dementias:

- Oily fish – once again, it's good for the brain
- Green and white tea – contains plant chemicals called catechins
- Fruit and vegetables – packed with antioxidants, which reduce damage to the brain by free-radical molecules
- Replace saturated fats (such as butter) with monounsaturated fats (such as olive oil)

Get Moving!

Being a couch potato really isn't healthy – our lack of exercise costs the NHS over one billion pounds a year! And a recent Oxford University study calculated that physical inactivity was directly responsible for 3 per cent of all deaths and illness. So much for the negative effects of not exercising – what about the positives for getting active? Well, think of the buzz that exercising provides, and the undeniable boost you'll get from looking fit and toned, and what more reason do you need to get moving?

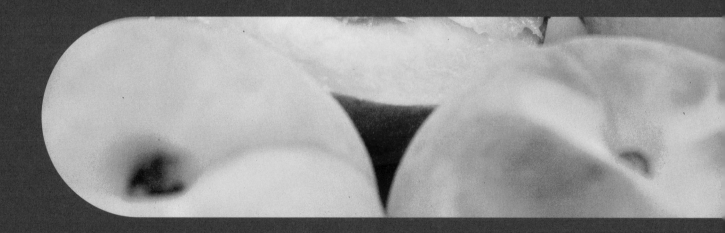

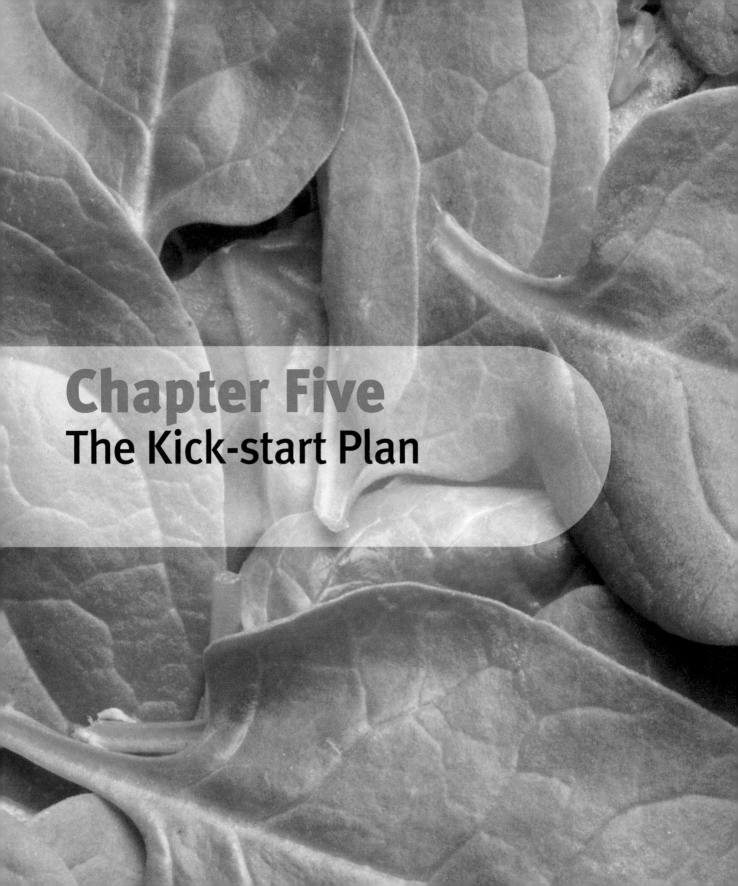

Chapter Five
The Kick-start Plan

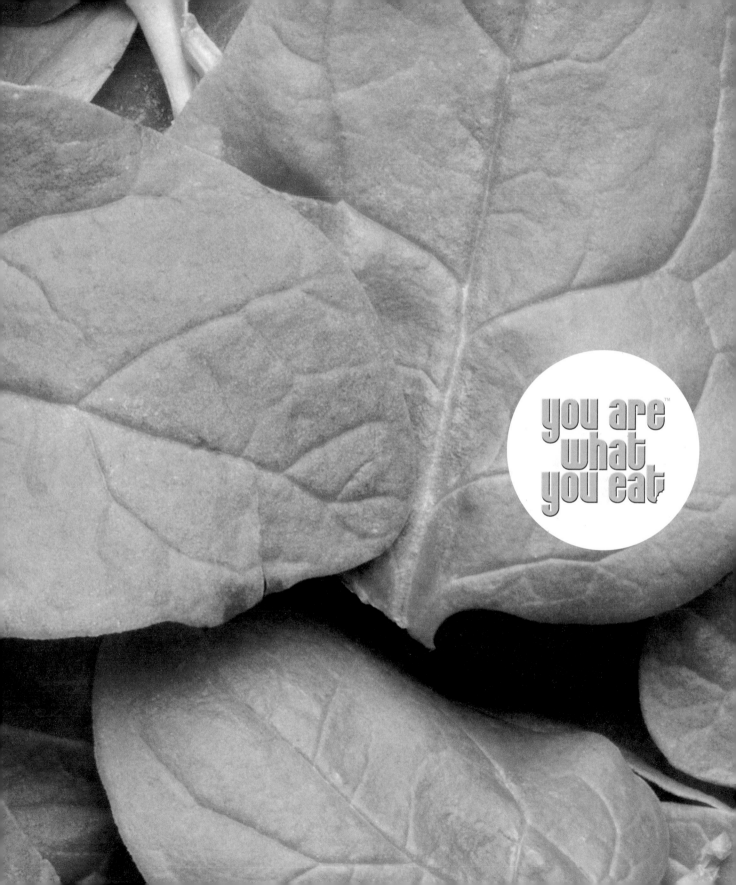

you are what you eat

The 28-day Kick-start plan

Now's the time to resolve to change your diet with our 28-day Kick-start Plan. It'll put you back on the straight and narrow if your good intentions have slipped, and get you into the You Are What You Eat healthy way of eating if you are a newcomer.

There is nothing difficult about the menu plan. You won't be expected to slave over a hot stove for hours on end or scour the high street for unfamiliar ingredients with unpronounceable names. Its main aim is to help you dump any junk from your diet and get you into the habit of eating a wide range of fresh vegetables and fruit, cut back on the sugar, salt and bad fats, and eat the kind of balanced diet that we all know we should be eating. It's not about self-denial but about changing your dietary lifestyle to boost your energy levels, reduce stress, and help keep you healthy.

In four weeks, you should be able to see and feel the benefits. You'll have lost some weight if you need to, and you'll have loads more energy. Plus, there will be the health changes you can't see – eating healthily can help to reduce your blood pressure, balance your blood sugar, and help you maintain healthy cholesterol levels.

It may seem difficult in the first few weeks, but if you stick to the plan it will help you break any bad old habits, encourage you to prepare quick and delicious meals from fresh ingredients and make healthy eating second nature to you.

If you're already at a healthy weight, and find that you're actually losing weight on the 28-day Kick-start Plan, increase the portions of the wholegrain carbohydrates (foods such as wholemeal bread, brown pasta, brown rice, etc.) slightly, and perhaps have slightly larger portions of protein foods such as fish, poultry, eggs and pulses. Also, have semi-skimmed milk rather than skimmed.

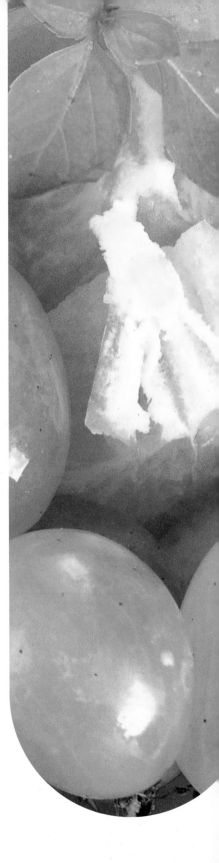

Use low-fat dairy products such as skimmed or semi-skimmed milk, and low-fat natural yogurt and fromage frais.

Top tips

- Ensure that you always eat at least two pieces of fruit and three portions of vegetables each day. It's a fabulous opportunity to try new and exotic fruits – fresh, frozen or tinned in juice – and any new vegetables. You don't need to stick to the fruits and vegetables listed in the menu plan – you can substitute alternatives.
- We've tried to vary the fruit in the plan, yet we don't want you to have to buy out-of-season fruits that have been flown or shipped halfway around the world. So, make the most of in-season fruit when you see it, and feel free to have this instead of the fruit in the plan. Just make sure you still get a good mixture of different kinds.
- Try to eat two portions of oily fish each week and one portion of white fish.
- If not stated in a recipe, portions of rice, pasta and noodles are 40g per person (uncooked weight).
- If not stated in a recipe, a portion of tinned fish is a small tin, a portion of fresh fish is approximately 150g, and a portion of meat or poultry is approximately 110g.
- For a spread, use one that is high in monounsaturates, such as olive spread, and use olive oil or canola oil in cooking. Always avoid spreads containing hydrogenated or partially hydrogenated oils, which are a source of harmful trans fats.
- In the menu plan, 'fruit spread' is the low-sugar high-fruit type that you have to keep in the fridge, not regular jam.
- Fresh fruit juice means pure fruit juice – not 'fruit juice drink' or squash.
- Always remove all visible fat and skin from meat and poultry. (You won't find red meat in the 28-day Kick-start Plan but don't worry, they return in the 'Forever Plan' when you'll also be ready to adapt your own favourite meals to incorporate into your new and healthy way of eating.)
- If during the weekend you prefer to have your main meal at lunchtime, feel free to swap the lunch and dinner menus.

You may well have bought books with eating plans before, and given up on them because you don't like the menu plans. We don't want you to do that with this book! Although our plan has been specially devised to give you all the nutrients you need, we realise that you may be intolerant to dairy products, for example, or a strict vegetarian. Or perhaps there's a certain food you just couldn't bear to eat – and it's in one of the recipes.

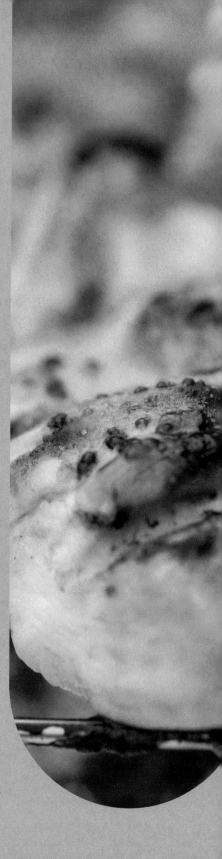

Just make the following simple changes:

- If you're a vegetarian, replace the non-vegetarian meals with those that are suitable. Once again, keep the variety as high as you can. To make sure you're absorbing enough iron, try to include some vitamin C-rich food with your meals, such as a small glass of orange juice.

- If you come across a menu suggestion that you really don't like, substitute a complete meal from another day.

- We've chosen vegetable accompaniments that complement the meals, both in terms of taste and nutrition, so give them a try. But if you really can't bear a particular vegetable, you can change it. Try to swap like for like, such as replacing one green vegetable with another.

- Even if you don't like a fruit or vegetable in the plan, give it a try. Only if you really don't like it, after trying it several times, substitute it for another. But make sure you're getting a wide variety of as many different kinds and colours of fruit and veg as possible. Be daring! If you stick to bananas and apples because that's what you've always liked, you'll be missing out on the nutritional benefits of all those exciting fruits out there.

Meat, Wheat and Dairy

You might be surprised to see foods such as meat, wheat and dairy products included in our healthy-eating plan. Several 'diets' ban these food groups, claiming that they produce toxins or are hard to digest.

As a consequence, many people remove these foods from their diet, thinking that this will make them feel better. In some cases, it may. If you go from eating a junk-food diet, and drastically cut out everything you've ever heard is 'bad', living only on non-wheat wholegrains, beans and pulses, fruit, vegetables and a little unsaturated oil, you probably will feel better than you did before, and may well lose weight. This will happen because you've cut out or reduced the unhealthy saturated fats, salt and sugar, and increased your healthy wholegrains, pulses, fruit and vegetables.

But we wouldn't recommend this kind of limited diet, for two main reasons:

- You could be in danger of becoming deficient in several important nutrients, such as protein, calcium, iron and vitamin B12

- Such a limited range of foods would make preparing meals and eating out very difficult, and you would be more likely to give up on your healthy-eating ideals as being too much effort

It is true that some people cannot eat dairy products or wheat or gluten-containing foods, because they are allergic to them, or have a severe intolerance. And some people avoid some or all meats or animal products for moral or religious reasons. These are all good reasons. But you shouldn't cut out these food groups simply to lose weight, because you think it's 'bad for you', and certainly not because you've read about it in the latest celebrity fad diet!

Am I allergic or intolerant?

As many as one in five people believe that they are intolerant or allergic to a particular food, but in fact less than 1 per cent of the UK's adult population have a true food allergy.

Although true food allergies are dangerous, and severe intolerances can make your life a misery, self-diagnosing these problems can leave your diet seriously lacking in vital nutrients.

Food allergies

If you have a food allergy, your body reacts to a food as if it is harmful, producing antibodies that trigger an allergic reaction, with immediate symptoms such as rashes, swelling, itchy skin, diarrhoea and other digestive upsets.

Anaphylaxis (or anaphylactic shock) is a particularly severe allergic reaction, where the airways swell, restricting breathing. This can be life-threatening, and people with this kind of food allergy must avoid the offending food. Their doctor will give them a special 'pen' to inject themselves with immediately they notice the symptoms, to open up the airways.

The most common food allergens are peanuts and other nuts, cows' milk, soya products (including soya milk), eggs, fish and shellfish, and wheat. Nuts account for most of the severe cases of food allergy.

Have you got a food allergy? The only reliable way of diagnosing a food allergy is to ask your doctor for an allergy test. If this is positive, he or she can then refer you to a dietician or other registered nutrition professional, to ensure that you still receive a balanced diet.

Food intolerances

The symptoms of food intolerances usually don't appear for hours or even days after eating. They include nausea, diarrhoea, stomach cramps, bloating and headaches.

Common food intolerances include milk, eggs, wheat, soya products, chocolate, caffeine, wine, some fruits, and some food additives.

Have you got a food intolerance? Far more people are intolerant to one or more foods than suffer from food allergy. Perhaps as many as 20 per cent of us have a food that 'disagrees with us', to a greater or lesser extent.

However, food intolerances are notoriously difficult to diagnose, and you shouldn't jump to conclusions or make assumptions that a particular food is behind your symptoms.

The symptoms of food intolerances are extremely variable, and don't appear until long after you've eaten the offending food, making the culprit hard to track down. There are no reliable scientific tests – the only way to diagnose intolerances is to remove the suspect food and see if symptoms reduce or disappear. You'd need to keep a food diary for several weeks.

If you plan to 'test-remove' any major food groups, such as dairy or wheat, you should ask your doctor to refer you to a registered nutrition professional for advice.

The Kick-start Plan

You'll find the recipes for meals marked with an asterisk (*) in Chapter 7.

The exercise part of the plan is aimed at complete beginners – you may well feel you can manage more. If so, that's great!

Please consult your doctor before starting any kind of diet or exercise plan if you are on any prescription medication, if you are a smoker, or are very overweight, or if you have any other health concerns.

WEEK 1

Build up your healthy store cupboard over the weeks, as you begin our healthy eating plan.

It may look a lot to buy, but you may find you have a lot of the storecupboard ingredients. And as you begin to build up your healthy store, you'll find the new ingredients you need become fewer and fewer. Then all you'll need to do is check your store cupboard regularly so you don't run out of your new healthy foods.

If you're not making some of the recipes, you'll find that you won't need everything on the lists below.

Week 1 store cupboard:

No-sugar no-salt muesli

Wholewheat bisks such as Weetabix

Wholemeal crispbreads

Porridge oats

Wholewheat pasta

Brown rice

Wholewheat noodles

Couscous

Tinned sweetcorn

Tinned salmon

Tinned borlotti or cannellini beans

Tinned chickpeas

Tinned tomatoes

Tinned low-sugar, low-salt baked beans

Tinned apricots

Small tins or pots fruit pieces in juice

Low-sugar fruit spread

Honey

Sultanas

Walnuts

Brazil nuts

Almonds

Hazel nuts

Mixed seeds (e.g. pumpkin, sunflower)

Ready-to-eat dried unsulphured apricots

Mild curry powder or paste

Dried mixed herbs

Chilli or harissa paste

Cumin

Cinnamon

Chilli powder

Ground black pepper

Salt

Low-calorie olive spray

Olive oil

Tomato purée

Worcestershire sauce

Soy sauce

Vegetable stock powder

Low-fat mayonnaise

Also check your fridge and freezer for:

Skimmed or semi-skimmed milk

Low-fat natural yogurt

Low-fat natural fromage frais

Low-fat cottage cheese with pineapple

Half-fat Cheddar cheese

Olive spread

Pure fruit juice

Frozen peas

Eggs

You should drink at least eight glasses (approximately 1.5 litres) of water each day of the plan.

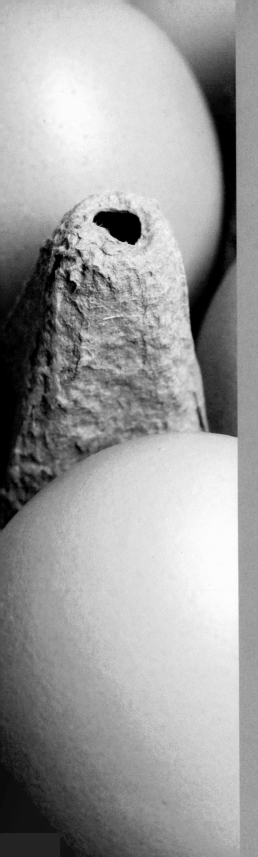

MONDAY

Breakfast: A serving of no-added-sugar or -salt muesli with skimmed or semi-skimmed milk or low-fat natural yogurt sweetened with a teaspoon of honey and topped with an individual pot of fruit pieces in juice. A small glass (110ml) of pure fruit juice.

Snack: An apple.

Lunch: A 150g pot of low-fat cottage cheese plus pineapple with a large bowl of mixed salad and four wholemeal crispbreads. A handful of grapes.

Snack: A pot of low-fat natural yogurt or fromage frais topped with a tablespoon of sultanas.

Dinner: *Baked Mango Chicken with Apple and Onion Raita, served with salad leaves and wholegrain rice. Two pineapple rings tinned in juice with two tablespoons low-fat natural yogurt or fromage frais.

EXERCISE A fifteen- to twenty-minute brisk walk (if you are walking briskly you should be able to talk but not sing!).

TUESDAY

Breakfast: A serving of porridge made with skimmed or semi-skimmed milk and sweetened with a teaspoon of sugar or honey. A banana. A small glass (110ml) of pure fruit juice.

Snack: Four ready-to-eat dried unsulphured apricots.

Lunch: A wholemeal ham and salad sandwich, four cherry tomatoes. A slice of malt loaf.

Snack: A large orange, or two satsumas, mandarins or clementines.

Dinner: *Sicilian Cod served with rice, green beans and broccoli. A low-fat natural yogurt topped with four chopped walnuts, a tablespoon of sultanas and a teaspoon of honey.

EXERCISE A fifteen- to twenty-minute brisk walk.

WEDNESDAY

Breakfast: A slice of wholemeal toast, spread with a little low-fat olive spread and low-sugar high-fruit spread. A small carton of low-fat natural yogurt topped with a handful of chopped nuts and seeds and sweetened with a teaspoon of honey. A small glass (110ml) of pure fruit juice.

Snack: A small banana.

Lunch: A wholemeal pitta bread filled with salad and tinned salmon with a dressing made with one teaspoon of yogurt and one teaspoon of low-fat mayonnaise. Two oatcakes spread with fruit spread.

Snack: A slice of malt loaf.

Dinner: *Vegetable Tagine with couscous (remember to reserve half for tomorrow's lunchtime salad). Three baked or poached pears served with two tablespoons of low-fat natural yogurt.

EXERCISE A fifteen- to twenty-minute brisk walk.

THURSDAY

Breakfast: Two Weetabix topped with four chopped, ready-to-eat, dried, unsulphured apricots and four prunes with semi-skimmed or skimmed milk. A small glass (110ml) of pure fruit juice.

Snack: A small banana.

Lunch: Vegetable Tagine (from yesterday's dinner) and couscous salad on a bed of lettuce. A pot of low-fat natural yogurt topped with a drizzle of honey and a tablespoon of nuts and seeds.

Snack: A tablespoon of sultanas and four walnut halves.

Dinner: *Mushroom and Egg Pan Fry, with new potatoes and sweetcorn. A baked peach sprinkled with cinnamon and served with two tablespoons of low-fat natural yogurt.

EXERCISE A fifteen- to twenty-minute brisk walk.

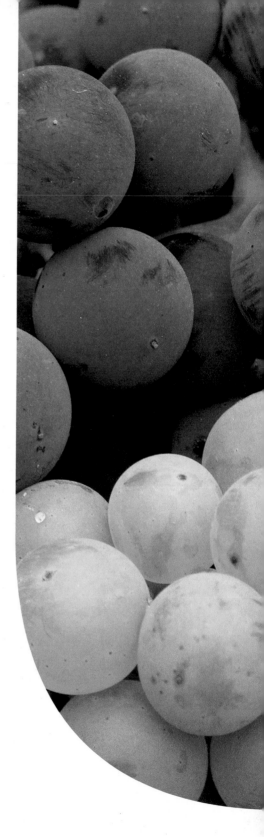

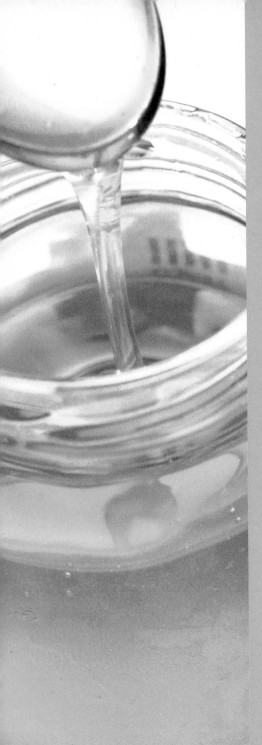

FRIDAY

Breakfast: A serving of porridge made with skimmed or semi-skimmed milk, topped with a chopped banana and a tablespoon of sultanas and sweetened with a teaspoon of honey, if needed. A small glass (110ml) of pure fruit juice.

Snack: An apple.

Lunch: A chicken and salad sandwich, a slice of malt loaf and a pot of small low-fat natural yogurt with chopped fresh or tinned fruit.

Snack: A peach or pear.

Dinner: *Tuna and Tomato Pasta with a large salad. A fruit fool made with a low-fat natural yogurt whizzed in a blender with a small tin of apricots (tinned in juice) and sprinkled with a tablespoon of nuts and seeds.

EXERCISE A fifteen- to twenty-minute brisk walk, plus a session of stretching/ flexibility exercises such as yoga or Pilates

SATURDAY

Breakfast: A tin of sardines, sprinkled with a little Worcestershire sauce, grilled on two slices of wholemeal toast, and a grilled tomato. A pear. A small glass (110ml) of semi-skimmed or skimmed milk.

Snack: A small banana.

Lunch: A jacket potato topped with a low-sugar/low-salt baked bean filling and a large salad.

Snack: A bunch of grapes.

Dinner: *Stir-fried Chicken with Broccoli served with wholegrain noodles. A mousse made by blending a small sliced mango with three tablespoons of low-fat natural yogurt.

EXERCISE A fifteen- to twenty-minute brisk walk or a twenty-minute swim.

SUNDAY

Breakfast: A toasted English muffin (preferably wholemeal) topped with two scrambled eggs and eight mushrooms, halved and sautéed in a little stock or water. A low-fat natural yogurt sweetened with a teaspoon of honey and topped with a teaspoon of chopped nuts. A small glass (110ml) of pure fruit juice.

Snack: A banana.

Lunch: *Hearty Bean Soup with crusty wholemeal bread.

Snack: A slice of malt loaf.

Dinner: *Oriental Salmon with new potatoes, a grilled tomato and green beans. A slice of melon.

EXERCISE A day off.

Week one notes

Why not keep a note of how you're feeling throughout the plan? Are there certain foods or meals you really enjoy? Are there some you really don't like? How do you feel as the weeks go on? It could act as a motivator to keep you on track to your ultimate goal of a fitter, healthier you. Altrnatively, make your own food diary – see page 218

Day/Time	Food	How do I feel?

WEEK 2

Week 2 store cupboard

Wholemeal self-raising flour
Brown plain flour
Baking powder
Bicarbonate of soda
Popping corn
Tinned tuna
Tinned butter beans
Wholegrain mustard
Sweet chilli dipping sauce
Balsamic vinegar
Paprika
Chilli powder
Black olives
Mild curry powder or paste

Also check your fridge and freezer for:

Skimmed or semi-skimmed milk
Low-fat natural yogurt
Low-fat natural fromage frais
Low-fat cottage cheese with pineapple
Low-fat plain cottage cheese
Half-fat Cheddar cheese
Pure fruit juice
Eggs
Low-fat cream cheese

MONDAY

Breakfast: A serving of wholegrain low-sugar cereal with skimmed or semi-skimmed milk. A slice of melon. A small glass (110ml) of pure fruit juice.

Snack: Veggie sticks (batons of carrot, celery, pepper, cucumber) with 2 tablespoons of *Healthy Hummus

Lunch: A tuna and salad filled wholemeal pitta bread. A pear.

Snack: A low-fat natural yogurt sweetened with honey and topped with a tablespoon of seeds.

Dinner: *Speedy Cheesy Spaghetti with a large green salad. A baked banana, drizzled with half a teaspoon of honey and sprinkled with a tablespoon of chopped nuts and two tablespoons of low-fat natural yogurt.

EXERCISE A fifteen- to twenty-minute brisk walk plus fifteen minutes of strength exercises.

TUESDAY

Breakfast: A serving of porridge made with skimmed or semi-skimmed milk, topped with a chopped banana and a tablespoon of sultanas and sweetened with a teaspoon of honey, if needed. A small glass (110ml) of pure fruit juice.

Snack: A kiwi fruit and four walnut halves.

Lunch: A 150g pot of low-fat cottage cheese with pineapple with a large bowl of mixed salad and four wholemeal crispbreads. An apple.

Snack: Two oatcakes and a handful of grapes.

Dinner: *Baked Chicken with Hot Mango and Pepper Salsa (keep some for tomorrow's lunch), served with a medium baked jacket potato and a large green salad. A low-fat natural fromage frais topped with a carton of fruit pieces in juice.

EXERCISE A fifteen- to twenty-minute brisk walk.

WEDNESDAY

Breakfast: 2 slices of wholemeal toast spread with a little low-fat olive spread. A fruit smoothie made with a small banana, half a mango, 110ml skimmed or semi-skimmed milk and three tablespoons of low-fat natural yogurt.

Snack: An apple.

Lunch: Baked sliced chicken breast (reserved from Tuesday's dinner) on a bed of salad, with a small wholemeal roll. A small low-fat natural yogurt with half a tin of peaches (tinned in juice) stirred in.

Snack: Five ready-to-eat, dried, unsulphured apricots.

Dinner: *Portuguese Fish with green beans and broccoli or new potatoes and a large green salad. A slice of melon.

EXERCISE A fifteen- to twenty-minute brisk walk plus fifteen minutes of strength exercises.

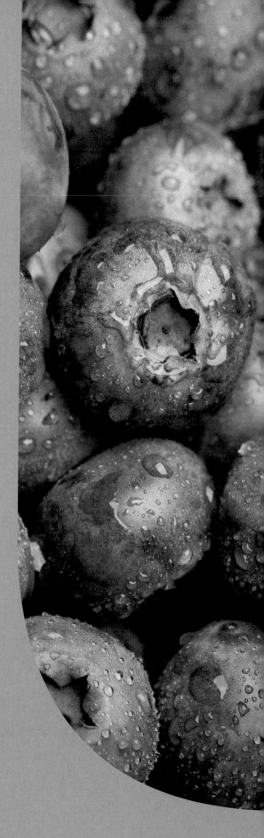

THURSDAY:

Breakfast: Two slices of fruit loaf toasted and spread with low-fat olive spread if you like. A small low-fat natural yogurt topped with a handful of berry fruits and a teaspoon of sunflower seeds. A small glass (110ml) of pure fruit juice.

Snack: Veggie sticks with two tablespoons of cottage cheese.

Lunch: A low-fat cream-cheese sandwich with watercress and a bowl of salad. A handful of grapes.

Snack: A slice of malt loaf.

Dinner: *Butter Bean and Vegetable Bake with green beans and broccoli or a large salad. Mango and apple fruit salad (made with half a mango and one chopped apple).

EXERCISE A fifteen- to twenty-minute brisk walk.

FRIDAY

Breakfast: A serving of porridge made with skimmed or semi-skimmed milk and sweetened with a teaspoon of honey. A banana. A small glass (110ml) of pure fruit juice.

Snack: An apple.

Lunch: A large bowl of salad topped with low-fat cottage cheese and served with a crusty wholemeal roll or four wholemeal crispbreads. An orange or a handful of grapes.

Snack: A low-fat natural yogurt topped with a tablespoon of sultanas and sweetened with a teaspoon of honey, if needed.

Dinner: *Grilled Salmon with Sweet Chilli Sauce on a bed of watercress with boiled new potatoes, green beans and a grilled tomato. Two wholemeal home-made *Scotch Pancakes topped with a handful of red berry fruits, two tablespoons of low-fat natural fromage frais and a drizzle of honey.

EXERCISE A fifteen- to twenty-minute brisk walk plus fifteen minutes of strength exercises.

SATURDAY

Breakfast: A slice of wholemeal toast topped with a small tin of reduced-sugar, reduced-salt baked beans and a grilled tomato. A pear. A small glass (110ml) of pure fruit juice.

Snack: A pot of plain home-popped popcorn (seasoned with a pinch of paprika or a little freshly ground black pepper, if liked).

Lunch: Cold grilled salmon served with a jacket or boiled potatoes and a large salad.

Snack: Five ready-to-eat, dried unsulphured apricots

Dinner: *Bean and Tomato Hotpot with Wholewheat Pasta and Broccoli. A poached pear with two tablespoons of low-fat natural fromage frais or natural yogurt.

EXERCISE A fifteen- to twenty-minute brisk walk or a twenty-minute swim.

SUNDAY

Breakfast: A wholemeal English muffin, toasted and topped with a poached egg, two rashers of lean grilled bacon and a grilled tomato. A small glass (110ml) of pure fruit juice.

Snack: An apple.

Lunch: A crusty wholemeal salmon and cucumber baguette and a large green salad. A slice of melon.

Snack: Two oatcakes spread with a little low-fat cream cheese.

Dinner: *Honey and Lemon Chicken with new potatoes and broccoli. A baked apple filled with one tablespoon of sultanas and two chopped walnuts.

EXERCISE A day off.

Week two notes

Day/Time	Food	How do I feel?

WEEK 3

MONDAY

Breakfast: Two Weetabix topped with four chopped, ready-to-eat, dried, unsulphured apricots and four prunes with semi-skimmed milk. A small glass (110ml) of pure fruit juice.

Snack: A small banana.

Lunch: A wholemeal sandwich filled with a sliced hard-boiled egg seasoned with freshly ground black pepper with lettuce, cucumber and tomato slices. A slice of malt loaf and a handful of grapes.

Snack: A low-fat natural yogurt topped with a tablespoon of sultanas and a drizzle of honey.

Dinner: *Spicy Pan-fried Fish with boiled new potatoes, sugar-snap peas and broccoli. A slice of melon.

EXERCISE A fifteen- to twenty-minute brisk walk plus fifteen minutes of strength exercises.

TUESDAY

Breakfast: A slice of wholemeal toast with low-fat olive spread. A natural yogurt topped with three chopped, ready-to-eat, dried, unsulphured apricots and three chopped walnut halves, sweetened with a half a teaspoon of honey, if needed. A small glass (110ml) of pure fruit juice.

Snack: A small banana.

Lunch: A chicken and wholemeal pasta salad on a bed of lettuce, four cherry tomatoes and a small crusty wholemeal roll. A low-fat natural yogurt with some chopped fresh fruit stirred in.

Snack: A pot of plain home-popped popcorn seasoned with a teaspoon of finely grated Parmesan cheese.

Dinner: *Salmon with Honey and Mustard served with new potatoes, green beans and broccoli or a large salad. A baked banana topped with chopped nuts, a drizzle of honey and two tablespoons of low-fat natural fromage frais.

EXERCISE A fifteen- to twenty-minute brisk walk.

WEDNESDAY

Breakfast: A serving of porridge made with skimmed or semi-skimmed milk, topped with a chopped banana and a tablespoon of sultanas and sweetened with a teaspoon of honey, if needed. A small glass (110ml) of pure fruit juice.

Snack: An apple.

Lunch: *Tuna and Bean Salad with a bed of lettuce and four wholemeal crispbreads or a crusty wholemeal roll. A handful of grapes.

Snack: A slice of malt loaf.

Dinner: *Quick Cajun Chicken Tortillas with a large green salad. A fresh fruit platter with two tablespoons of low-fat natural yogurt and a drizzle of honey.

EXERCISE A fifteen- to twenty-minute brisk walk plus fifteen minutes of strength exercises.

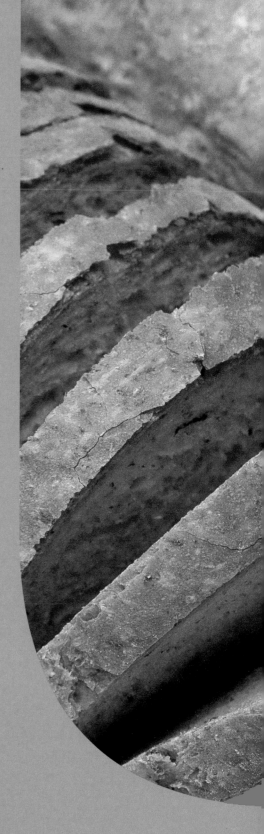

THURSDAY

Breakfast: A serving of no-added-sugar or -salt muesli with milk or low-fat natural yogurt and topped with an individual carton or pot of fruit pieces in juice. A small glass (110ml) of pure fruit juice.

Snack: A banana.

Lunch: Chicken wrap (home-made using healthy ingredients, or bought from a 'healthy' range) accompanied by a green salad. A slice of malt loaf. A low-fat natural yogurt or fromage frais with some chopped fresh fruit stirred in.

Snack: Two oatcakes spread with a little low-fat cream cheese.

Dinner: *Spicy Baked Beans served with wholegrain rice or pasta and green vegetables and a large green salad. A handful of grapes.

EXERCISE A fifteen- to twenty-minute brisk walk.

FRIDAY

Breakfast: Two slices of wholemeal toast with peanut butter or fruit spread. A pear. A small glass (110ml) of semi-skimmed milk.

Snack: A small banana.

Lunch: A wholemeal salmon and cucumber sandwich. Four cherry tomatoes. A handful of blueberries.

Snack: A slice of malt loaf.

Dinner: *Pasta with Feta Cubes served with a large green salad. Four baked plums with two tablespoons of low-fat natural yogurt or fromage frais and a drizzle of honey.

EXERCISE A fifteen- to twenty-minute brisk walk plus fifteen minutes of strength exercises.

SATURDAY

Breakfast: A slice of wholemeal toast topped with a small tin of reduced-sugar, reduced-salt baked beans and a grilled tomato. A pear. A small glass (110ml) of pure fruit juice.

Snack: An apple.

Lunch: *Seafood Pizza served with a large salad.

Snack: A pot of plain home-popped popcorn flavoured with a teaspoon of Parmesan cheese.

Dinner: *Bean Stew with new potatoes, cabbage and broccoli. A baked peach with two tablespoons of low-fat natural yogurt.

EXERCISE A fifteen- to twenty-minute brisk walk or a twenty-minute swim.

SUNDAY

Breakfast: A mushroom omelette with grilled tomatoes. A slice of wholemeal toast with low-fat olive spread and low-sugar marmalade. A handful of grapes. A small glass (110ml) of pure fruit juice.

Snack: An apple or orange.

Lunch: A medium baked jacket potato filled with reduced-sugar, reduced-salt baked beans and served with a large green salad.

Snack: A low-fat natural yogurt topped with a tablespoon of sultanas and a little honey to sweeten.

Dinner: *Mustard and Rosemary Roast Chicken with Baby Roast Potatoes, with carrots and broccoli or cabbage. Fresh fruit salad topped with two tablespoons of low-fat natural fromage frais and a tablespoon of chopped nuts.

EXERCISE A day off.

Week three notes

Day/Time	Food	How do I feel?

WEEK 4

Week 4 store cupboard:
Tinned pineapple in juice
Dried or frozen basil
Dried or frozen parsley
Dried or frozen rosemary
Garlic flakes

Also check your fridge and freezer for:
Low-fat natural yogurt
Low-fat natural fromage frais
Low-fat cottage cheese with pineapple
Skimmed or semi-skimmed milk
Olive spread
Half-fat Cheddar cheese
Parmesan
Pure fruit juice
Eggs
Frozen peas

MONDAY

Breakfast: A slice of wholemeal toast, spread with a little low-fat olive spread and fruit spread. A small carton of low-fat natural yogurt topped with a handful of chopped nuts and seeds and sweetened with a teaspoon of honey. A small glass (110ml) of pure fruit juice.

Snack: A banana.

Lunch: A salmon, tuna or prawn wholemeal pasta salad. A handful of grapes.

Snack: A slice of malt loaf.

Dinner: *Chicken Stir-fry with Chinese Leaves and noodles. Three pineapple rings (tinned in juice) with two tablespoons of low-fat natural fromage frais.

EXERCISE A thirty-minute brisk walk plus twenty minutes of strength exercises.

TUESDAY

Breakfast: A serving of no-added-sugar or -salt muesli with milk or low-fat natural yogurt topped with an individual carton or pot of fruit pieces in juice. A small glass (110ml) of pure fruit juice.

Snack: Small handful of grapes.

Lunch: A lean ham and salad wholemeal sandwich or wrap. Four cherry tomatoes. A slice of malt loaf. A pear.

Snack: A pot of plain home-popped popcorn flavoured with a teaspoon of grated Parmesan cheese.

Dinner: *Chickpea Chilli with brown rice and a large salad. Two *Scotch Pancakes with a small mango puréed and two tablespoons of low-fat natural fromage frais.

EXERCISE A thirty-minute brisk walk.

WEDNESDAY

Breakfast: Two Weetabix topped with four chopped, ready-to-eat, dried, unsulphured apricots and four prunes with skimmed or semi-skimmed milk. A small glass (110ml) of pure fruit juice.

Snack: An apple.

Lunch: A wholemeal pitta bread filled with tinned salmon and salad. A handful of grapes.

Snack: Two *Scotch Pancakes.

Dinner: *Baked Fish with Cheesy Crumb Topping, new potatoes, peas, sweetcorn and grilled tomatoes.

EXERCISE A thirty-minute brisk walk plus twenty minutes of strength exercises.

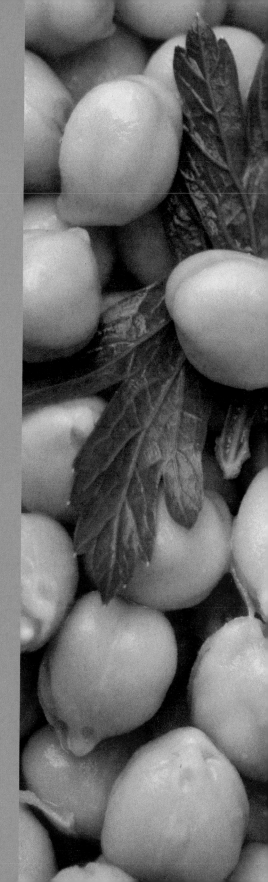

THURSDAY

Breakfast: A serving of porridge made with skimmed or semi-skimmed milk, topped with a chopped banana and a tablespoon of sultanas and sweetened with a teaspoon of honey, if needed. A small glass (110ml) of pure fruit juice.

Snack: An apple.

Lunch: A 150g pot of low-fat cottage cheese with pineapple, a portion of vegetable sticks – carrot, pepper, celery, cucumber – and four wholemeal crispbreads. A pear or a handful of grapes.

Snack: A slice of malt loaf.

Dinner: *Chicken and Bean Curry with brown basmati rice and salad. A pear poached in orange juice with two tablespoons of low-fat natural yogurt or fromage frais.

EXERCISE A thirty-minute brisk walk plus twenty minutes of strength exercises.

FRIDAY

Breakfast: A wholemeal English muffin toasted and spread with low-fat olive spread and low-sugar fruit jam or fruit spread. A small low-fat natural yogurt topped with a handful of berry fruits and a teaspoon of sunflower seeds. A small glass (110ml) of pure fruit juice.

Snack: A pot of plain home-popped popcorn flavoured with a pinch of paprika or a teaspoon of Parmesan cheese.

Lunch: A chicken and salad sandwich and four cherry tomatoes. Two *Scotch Pancakes spread with a little fruit spread.

Snack: A peach or pear.

Dinner: *Mediterranean Prawns and Pasta. A baked apple stuffed with a tablespoon of sultanas and chopped nuts, served with two tablespoons of low-fat fromage frais.

EXERCISE A thirty-minute brisk walk plus twenty minutes of strength exercises.

SATURDAY

Breakfast: A tin of sardines, sprinkled with a little Worcestershire sauce, grilled on two slices of wholemeal toast, and a grilled tomato. A pear. A small glass (110ml) of semi-skimmed milk.

Snack: Six cherry tomatoes.

Lunch: *Spanish Omelette with a wholemeal crusty roll. A low-fat natural yogurt with a tablespoon of raisins.

Snack: A slice of malt loaf or two *Scotch Pancakes, spread with fruit spread and sandwiched together.

Dinner: *Healthy Home-made Fish and Chips, with peas, sweetcorn and grilled tomato. A low-fat natural yogurt topped with a handful of crushed blueberries and a drizzle of honey.

EXERCISE A thirty-minute brisk walk or a thirty-minute swim or cycle.

SUNDAY

Breakfast: A toasted English muffin (preferably wholemeal) topped with two scrambled eggs, eight mushrooms, halved and sautéed in a little stock or water and a grilled tomato. A small glass (110ml) of pure fruit juice.

Snack: A banana.

Lunch: *Home-made Ham, Pineapple and Sweetcorn Pizza with a large salad.

Snack: A low-fat natural yogurt topped with red berry fruits and sweetened with a little honey if needed.

Dinner: *Sweet-and-sour Chicken Stir-fry with brown rice.

EXERCISE A day off.

Week four notes

Day/Time	Food	How do I feel?

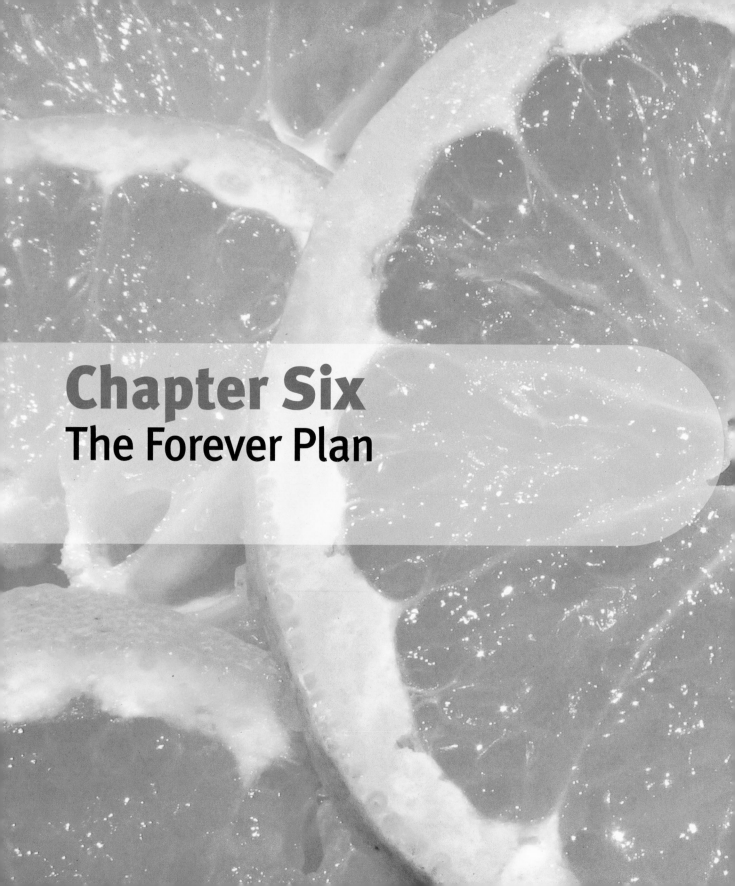

Chapter Six
The Forever Plan

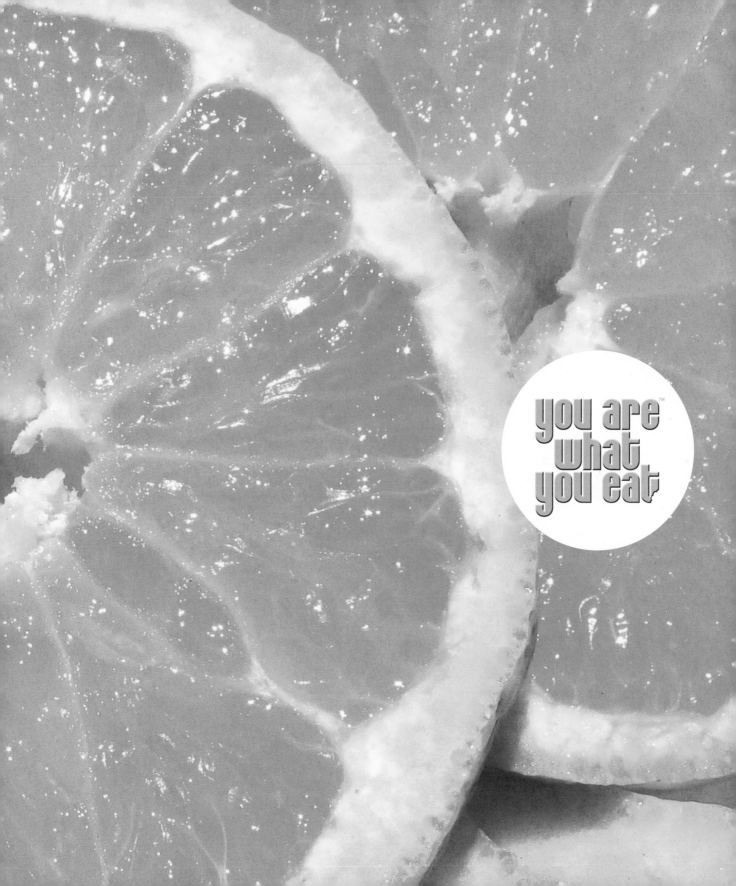

you are what you eat™

The Next Step

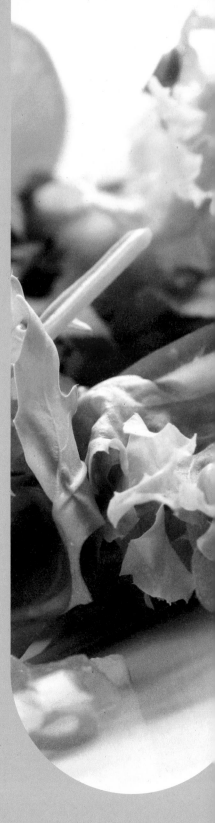

Now that you've mastered our fresh, healthy-eating philosophy, you can become more adventurous and flexible, devise your own healthy meals and adapt your family favourites. To get you started we've devised a 28-day menu plan full of delicious, speedy and fresh ideas. Please give them a try – it will help to increase your meal repertoire.

Eating healthily doesn't mean that you can't enjoy sharing meals with friends or visiting restaurants and coffee shops. You just need to make wise choices and learn how food on the menu is likely to have been prepared and what the dishes may contain. Don't be embarrassed if you don't know – ask the waiter. Become familiar with the cooking methods used in ethnic restaurants and skip any dishes that include rich sauces, cream, are heavily salted or sweetened, or have been fried.

There's no need to say goodbye to such favourites as burgers and pizzas and even chips. It's simple to prepare your own home-made, fresh, healthy versions. And if you fall off the wagon from time to time, it's not a major disaster. If you eat healthily 90 per cent of the time, the remaining 10 per cent of less than healthy choices won't do you any harm. There has to be room in life for treats.

Here are some tips to help you choose meals you can enjoy when you're out and about, without falling off the healthy-eating wagon:

- Skip the starters or settle for a slice of melon, grapefruit, a clear soup or a small salad without dressing as your starter
- Take a glance at the meals of fellow diners – if the portions are larger than you would like ask for a 'starter size' portion and a double-sized serving of vegetables and a side salad
- Ask for vegetables to be served without dressings or butter
- Ask if sauces can be served separately so you can use as little as you need
- When having coffee, go for 'skinny' versions and skip the syrups, cream and marshmallows

As you begin planning your own menus, try to make these simple guidelines a way of life:

- Include at least five portions of fruit and vegetables a day
- Use wholemeal bread, rice, noodles and pasta in place of white
- Eat red meat only once or twice a week
- Include oily fish twice a week, and white fish once a week
- Use skimmed or semi-skimmed milk, and other low-fat dairy products
- Try to have vegetarian meals or meals containing beans and pulses at least twice a week (always read the labels and select products that are low-fat, low-sugar and low-salt)
- Drink at least eight to ten glasses of water each day

Again, you'll find the recipes for meals marked with an asterisk (*) in Chapter 7.

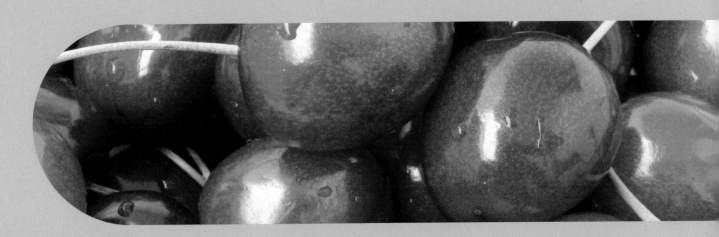

WEEK 1

Week 1 Store cupboard
Continental or puy lentils
Chilli flakes
Turmeric

Also check your fridge and freezer for:
Low-fat natural yogurt
Low-fat natural fromage frais
Low-fat cottage cheese
Skimmed or semi-skimmed milk
Olive spread
Half-fat Cheddar cheese
Feta or mozzarella cheese
Pure fruit juice
Eggs
Frozen peas

MONDAY

Breakfast: A serving of porridge made with skimmed or semi-skimmed milk and sweetened with a teaspoon of honey. A banana. A small glass (110ml) of pure fruit juice.

Snack: An apple, two oatcakes.

Lunch: *Vegetable Tagine and couscous salad on a bed of lettuce.

Snack: A yogurt pot filled with plain (home-popped) popcorn.

Dinner: *Speedy Cheesy Spaghetti with a large salad. A baked apple stuffed with one tablespoon of sultanas and served with two tablespoons of low-fat natural yogurt.

EXERCISE A thirty-minute brisk walk, or fifteen minutes' brisk walking plus fifteen minutes' jogging.

TUESDAY

Breakfast: A serving of no-added-sugar or -salt muesli with semi-skimmed or skimmed milk or low-fat natural yogurt sweetened with a teaspoon of honey and topped with an individual pot of fruit pieces in juice. A small glass (110ml) of pure fruit juice.

Snack: A banana.

Lunch: A wholemeal ham and salad sandwich, four cherry tomatoes and a slice of malt loaf.

Snack: An orange and a *Raisin Rock Cake.

Dinner: *Baked Chilli Chicken and Fruity Rice Salad. A bowl of strawberries topped with two tablespoons of low-fat fromage frais.

EXERCISE A thirty-minute brisk walk plus twenty minutes of strength exercises.

WEDNESDAY

Breakfast: A slice of wholemeal toast spread with a little low-fat olive spread. A fruit smoothie made with a small banana, half a mango, 110ml skimmed or semi-skimmed milk and three tablespoons of low-fat natural yogurt.

Snack: A small banana, two oatcakes.

Lunch: One slice of lean ham, a hard-boiled egg, six cherry tomatoes, a large green salad and a wholemeal roll lightly spread with low-fat olive spread. A pear.

Snack: An apple.

Dinner: *Baked Portuguese Cod with Sweetcorn Mash and Green Beans, with broccoli. A low-fat natural yogurt topped with four chopped walnuts, a tablespoon of sultanas and a teaspoon of honey.

EXERCISE An aerobic exercise or dance class.

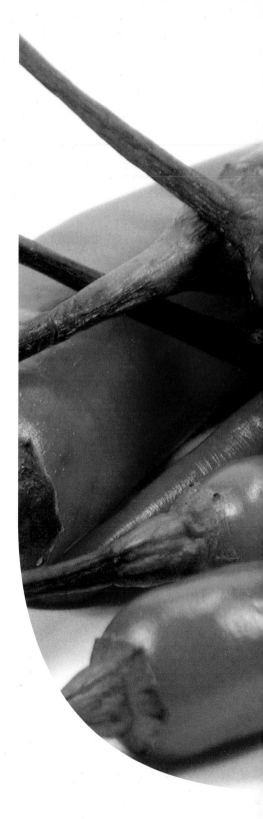

THURSDAY

Breakfast: Two Weetabix topped with four chopped, ready-to-eat, dried, unsulphured apricots and four prunes with skimmed or semi-skimmed milk. A small glass (110ml) of pure fruit juice.

Snack: A small banana.

Lunch: A wholemeal pitta bread filled with salad and tinned salmon. A small low-fat natural yogurt. A peach or two plums.

Snack: An apple and a *Raisin Rock Cake.

Dinner: *Baked Chicken with Hot Mango and Pepper Salsa, served with a medium baked jacket potato and a large green salad. A low-fat natural fromage frais topped with a sliced peach or a pot of fruit pieces in juice.

EXERCISE A thirty-minute brisk walk, swim or cycle, plus twenty minutes of strength exercises.

FRIDAY

Breakfast: A serving of porridge made with skimmed or semi-skimmed milk, topped with a chopped banana and a tablespoon of sultanas, and sweetened with a teaspoon of honey, if needed. A small glass (110ml) of pure fruit juice.

Snack: An apple and an oatcake.

Lunch: A large bowl of salad topped with low-fat cottage cheese and served with a crusty wholemeal roll or four wholemeal crispbreads. An orange or a handful of grapes.

Snack: A pear and a *Raisin Rock Cake.

Dinner: *Glazed Tuna Steak with New Potatoes and a Large Mixed Salad. A *Baked Fruit Parcel with two tablespoons of low-fat natural fromage frais.

EXERCISE: A thirty-minute brisk walk, or fifteen minutes' brisk walking plus fifteen minutes' jogging.

SATURDAY

Breakfast: A tin of sardines, sprinkled with a little Worcestershire sauce, grilled on two small slices of wholemeal toast, and a grilled tomato. A pear. A small glass (110ml) of semi-skimmed or skimmed milk.

Snack: A small banana and a yogurt pot filled with plain popcorn.

Lunch: A jacket potato with a tinned salmon or tuna and sweetcorn filling or a tuna and sweetcorn sandwich (wholemeal bread) and a large salad.

Snack: An apple and small wholemeal currant bun.

Dinner: *Curried Lentil Bake with a large mixed salad and cucumber raita. Two pineapple rings in juice, four chopped walnuts and two tablespoons of low-fat natural yogurt.

EXERCISE 30 minutes' swimming or a yoga, martial arts or relaxation class.

SUNDAY

Breakfast: A toasted wholemeal English muffin topped with scrambled egg and eight mushrooms, halved and sautéed in a little stock or water. A low-fat natural yogurt sweetened with a teaspoon of honey and topped with a teaspoon of chopped nuts. A small glass (110ml) of pure fruit juice.

Snack: A banana.

Lunch: Spicy chicken wrap (healthy bought version, or try our *Quick Cajun Chicken Tortillas, served cold) accompanied by a green salad. A slice of malt loaf. A low-fat natural yogurt with chopped fresh fruit or a tablespoon of dried fruit.

Snack: An orange or four cherry tomatoes.

Dinner: *Honeyed Lamb Chops with mashed potatoes, carrots and green beans. Poached pear with 2 tablespoons of low-fat natural fromage frais or natural yogurt.

EXERCISE A thirty-minute brisk walk, swim or cycle, plus twenty minutes of strength exercises.

Week one notes

Day/Time	Food	How do I feel?

WEEK 2

Store cupboard:
Tinned crab
Black treacle
Cajun seasoning

Also check your fridge and freezer for:
Low-fat natural yogurt
Low-fat natural fromage frais
Low-fat cottage cheese
Low-fat cream cheese
Low-fat crème fraiche
Skimmed or semi-skimmed milk
Olive spread
Half-fat mature Cheddar cheese
Pure fruit juice
Eggs

MONDAY

Breakfast: One large egg, scrambled, a large portion of sliced mushrooms sautéed in stock or water, with a slice of wholemeal toast (served with the egg and mushrooms, or spread with one teaspoon of low-sugar marmalade). A pear. A small glass (110ml) of skimmed or semi-skimmed milk.

Snack: Veggie sticks (carrot, celery, pepper, cucumber) with two tablespoons of *Healthy Hummus.

Lunch: A wholemeal pitta bread filled with salad and tinned salmon and a dressing made with one teaspoon of yogurt and one teaspoon of low-fat mayonnaise. Two oatcakes spread with fruit spread.

Snack: A low-fat natural yogurt sweetened with honey and topped with a tablespoon of seeds.

Dinner: *Crab and Tomato Pasta with a large green salad. A sliced mango with two tablespoons of low-fat natural fromage frais topped with a tablespoon of chopped nuts and seeds.

EXERCISE A thirty-minute brisk walk, or fifteen minutes' brisk walking plus fifteen minutes' jogging.

TUESDAY

Breakfast: A serving of porridge made with skimmed or semi-skimmed milk, topped with a chopped banana and a tablespoon of sultanas and sweetened with a teaspoon of honey, if needed. A small glass (110ml) of pure fruit juice.

Snack: A kiwi fruit and four walnut halves.

Lunch: One slice of lean ham, a hard-boiled egg, six cherry tomatoes, a large green salad and a wholemeal roll lightly spread with low-fat olive spread. A pear.

Snack: A slice of malt loaf and a bunch of grapes.

Dinner: A chicken breast sprinkled with Cajun seasoning and baked in a foil parcel, served with boiled or steamed new potatoes, broccoli and green beans. A low-fat fruit yogurt.

EXERCISE A thirty-minute brisk walk, plus twenty minutes of strength exercises.

WEDNESDAY

Breakfast: A slice of wholemeal toast, spread with a little low-fat olive spread and fruit spread. A small carton of low-fat natural yogurt topped with a handful of chopped nuts and seeds and sweetened with a teaspoon of honey. A small glass (110ml) of pure fruit juice.

Snack: An apple and a small carton of plain popcorn.

Lunch: Sliced roast chicken breast on a bed of salad, with a small wholemeal roll. A low-fat natural yogurt with a handful of berry fruits stirred in.

Snack: Three ready-to-eat, dried, unsulphured apricots and a *Scotch Pancake.

Dinner: *Butter Bean and Vegetable Bake with green beans and broccoli or a large salad. Mango and apple fruit salad (made with half a mango and one chopped apple).

EXERCISE An aerobic exercise class or dance class.

THURSDAY

Breakfast: A toasted wholemeal English muffin spread with fruit spread. A low-fat natural yogurt topped with a handful of berry fruits and a tablespoon of sunflower seeds. A small glass (110ml) of pure fruit juice.

Snack: Veggie sticks with two tablespoons of cottage cheese.

Lunch: A low-fat cream-cheese sandwich (wholemeal bread) with watercress and a bowl of salad. A handful of grapes.

Snack: Two *Scotch Pancakes and a bunch of grapes.

Dinner: *Grilled Fish and Spicy Lentils, with boiled new potatoes, mangetout and grilled tomatoes. A *Baked Fruit Parcel topped with two tablespoons of low-fat natural fromage frais.

EXERCISE A thirty-minute brisk walk, swim or cycle, plus twenty minutes of strength exercises.

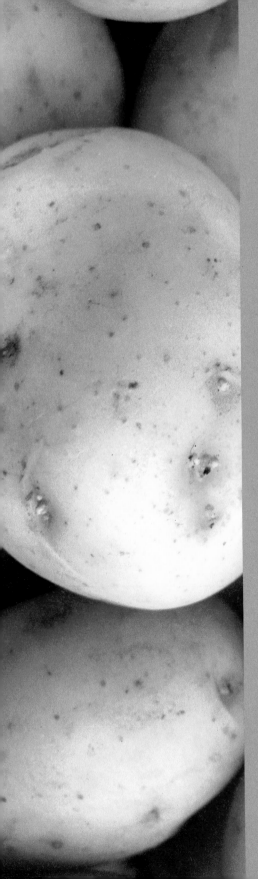

FRIDAY

Breakfast: A serving of porridge made with skimmed or semi-skimmed milk and sweetened with a teaspoon of honey. A banana. A small glass (110ml) of pure fruit juice.

Snack: An apple and three Brazil nuts.

Lunch: One slice of lean ham, a hard-boiled egg, six cherry tomatoes, a large green salad and a wholemeal roll lightly spread with low-fat olive spread. A pear, peach or nectarine.

Snack: A low-fat natural yogurt topped with a tablespoon of sultanas and a drizzle of honey.

Dinner: *Grilled Salmon with Sweet Chilli Sauce on a bed of watercress with boiled new potatoes, green beans and a grilled tomato. A fresh fruit platter served with two tablespoons of low-fat natural fromage frais.

EXERCISE A thirty-minute brisk walk, or fifteen minutes' brisk walking plus fifteen minutes' jogging.

SATURDAY

Breakfast: A slice of wholemeal toast topped with a small tin of reduced-sugar, reduced-salt baked beans and a grilled tomato. A pear. A small glass (110ml) of pure fruit juice.

Snack: A handful of grapes and a pot of plain popcorn (seasoned with a pinch of paprika or a little freshly ground black pepper, if liked).

Lunch: *Baked Bean Chowder and Wholemeal Soda Bread. A low-fat natural yogurt with one teaspoon of honey and one tablespoon of chopped walnuts. A handful of blueberries or other berries.

Snack: Two *Scotch Pancakes and three dried, ready-to-eat, unsulphured apricots.

Dinner: *Stir-fried Beef with Broccoli served with wholewheat noodles. A mousse made by blending a small sliced mango with three tablespoons of low-fat natural yogurt.

EXERCISE Thirty minutes' swimming or a yoga, martial arts or relaxation class.

SUNDAY

Breakfast: A wholemeal English muffin, toasted and topped with a poached egg, two rashers of lean grilled bacon, and a grilled tomato. A small glass (110ml) of pure fruit juice.

Snack: An apple and three walnut halves.

Lunch: Cream cheese, salmon and watercress wholemeal bagel. A slice of melon.

Snack: Two oatcakes spread with a little low-fat cream cheese.

Dinner: *Tomato Topped Chicken with Warm Herby Potatoes and a Green Salad. A slice of melon with a handful of red berries.

EXERCISE A thirty-minute brisk walk, swim or cycle, plus twenty minutes of strength exercises.

Week two notes

Day/Time	Food	How do I feel?

WEEK 3

Store cupboard:
Tinned Butter beans
Tinned Red kidney beans
Low-fat olive spread

Also check your fridge and freezer for:
Low-fat natural yogurt
Low-fat natural fromage frais
Semi-skimmed or skimmed milk
Low-fat cottage cheese with pineapple
Low-fat crème fraiche
Half-fat mature Cheddar cheese
Parmesan cheese
Olive spread
Pure fruit juice
Eggs

MONDAY

Breakfast: Two Weetabix topped with four chopped, ready-to-eat, dried, unsulphured apricots and four prunes with skimmed or semi-skimmed milk. A small glass (110ml) of pure fruit juice.

Snack: A small banana.

Lunch: A wholemeal sandwich filled with a sliced hard-boiled egg seasoned with freshly ground black pepper with lettuce, cucumber and tomato slices. A slice of malt loaf and a handful of grapes.

Snack: A low-fat natural yogurt topped with a tablespoon of sultanas and a drizzle of honey, if needed.

Dinner: *Mushroom and Broccoli Pasta with a large salad. Three baked plums with a tablespoon of low-sugar muesli and two tablespoons of low-fat natural fromage frais or yogurt.

EXERCISE A thirty-minute brisk walk, swim or cycle, plus twenty minutes of strength exercises.

TUESDAY

Breakfast: A slice of wholemeal toast with low-fat olive spread. A low-fat natural yogurt topped with three chopped, dried, unsulphured apricots and three chopped walnut halves, sweetened with half a teaspoon of honey, if needed. A small glass (110ml) of pure fruit juice.

Snack: A small banana.

Lunch: *Tuna and Bean Salad with a bed of lettuce and four wholemeal crispbreads or a crusty wholemeal roll. A handful of grapes.

Snack: A pot of plain popcorn seasoned with a teaspoon of finely grated Parmesan cheese.

Dinner: *Cauliflower and Butter Bean Curry with Mint Raita and brown rice. *Baked Fruit Parcels with two tablespoons of low-fat natural fromage frais.

EXERCISE Thirty minutes' brisk walking and jogging or thirty minutes' cycling or swimming.

WEDNESDAY

Breakfast: A serving of porridge made with skimmed or semi-skimmed milk, topped with a chopped banana and a tablespoon of sultanas and sweetened with a teaspoon of honey, if needed. A small glass (110ml) of pure fruit juice.

Snack: An apple and a pot of plain popcorn.

Lunch: One slice of roast chicken, a hard-boiled egg, six cherry tomatoes, a large green salad and a wholemeal roll lightly spread with low-fat olive spread. A pear or kiwi fruit.

Snack: A peach, nectarine or orange and a slice of malt loaf.

Dinner: *Grilled Fish and Spicy Lentils, with sugar-snap peas, broccoli and grilled tomato. A slice of melon and a handful of red berries.

EXERCISE An aerobic exercise or dance class.

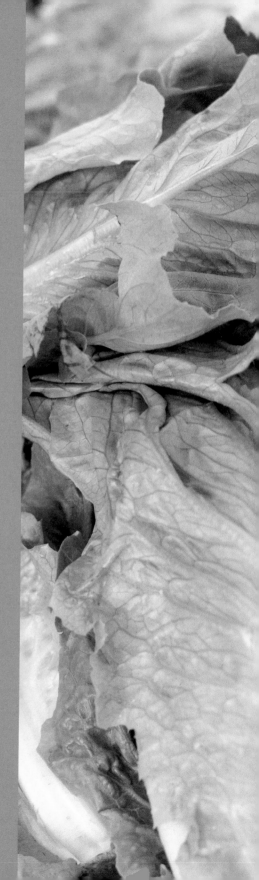

THURSDAY

Breakfast: A serving of no-added-sugar or -salt muesli with skimmed or semi-skimmed milk. A low-fat natural yogurt, served on the muesli, or sweetened with a teaspoon of honey and topped with an individual pot of fruit pieces in juice. A small glass (110ml) of pure fruit juice.

Snack: A banana or a peach.

Lunch: A 150g pot of low-fat cottage cheese with pineapple, with a large bowl of mixed salad and four wholemeal crispbreads. An apple.

Snack: Two oatcakes spread with a little low-fat cream cheese.

Dinner: *Vegetable Pasta with a large salad. A low-fat fruit yogurt and a piece of fruit.

EXERCISE A thirty-minute brisk walk, swim or cycle, plus twenty minutes of strength exercises.

FRIDAY

Breakfast: A bowl of no-sugar-added wholewheat cereal with a piece of fruit and a low-fat natural yogurt. A small glass (110ml) of pure fruit juice.

Snack: A small banana or an apple.

Lunch: A wholemeal salmon and cucumber sandwich, four cherry tomatoes and a slice of malt loaf. A peach or nectarine.

Snack: A portion of veggie sticks with two tablespoons of *Healthy Hummus.

Dinner: *Honey and Lemon Chicken with new potatoes, sweetcorn and broccoli. A tropical fruit salad platter – pineapple, lychee, banana – with two tablespoons of low-fat fromage frais.

EXERCISE A thirty-minute brisk walk, jog, swim or cycle.

SATURDAY

Breakfast: A slice of wholemeal toast topped with a small tin of reduced-sugar, reduced-salt baked beans and a grilled tomato. A pear. A small glass (110ml) of pure fruit juice.

Snack: A *Wholemeal Scone spread with a little fruit spread or low-fat olive spread.

Lunch: *Hearty Bean Soup with home-made *Wholemeal Soda Bread or a crusty wholemeal roll.

Snack: An apple and a pot of plain popcorn flavoured with a teaspoon of Parmesan cheese.

Dinner: *Glazed Salmon with Warm Orange and Mango Salsa, new potatoes, green beans and mangetout. A baked apple filled with one tablespoon of sultanas, three chopped walnuts and two tablespoons of low-fat natural fromage frais.

EXERCISE Forty minutes' swimming or a yoga, martial arts or relaxation class.

SUNDAY

Breakfast: A mushroom omelette with grilled tomatoes. A slice of wholemeal toast with low-fat olive spread and low-sugar marmalade. A handful of grapes. A small glass (110ml) of pure fruit juice.

Snack: An apple or orange and a *Wholemeal Scone spread with a little fruit spread.

Lunch: Chicken and wholemeal pasta salad with a crusty wholemeal roll. A low-fat natural yogurt topped with a chopped pear.

Week three notes

Snack: A slice of malt loaf and a handful of grapes.

Dinner: A grilled lamb chop (fat removed) with sweetcorn mash, a baked tomato, green beans and broccoli. Fresh fruit salad topped with two tablespoons of low-fat natural yogurt, a drizzle of honey and a tablespoon of seeds.

EXERCISE: A thirty-minute brisk walk, swim or cycle, plus twenty minutes of strength exercises.

Day/Time	Food	How do I feel?

Week 4

Week 4 storecupboard
Dijon or mild mustard

Also check your fridge and freezer for:
Semi-skimmed or skimmed milk
Low-fat natural yogurt
Low-fat natural fromage frais
Pure fruit juice
Olive spread
Parmesan cheese
Eggs
Low-fat cottage cheese
Cooked frozen prawns

MONDAY

Breakfast: A slice of wholemeal toast, spread with a little low-fat olive spread and fruit spread. A low-fat natural yogurt topped with a tablespoonful of chopped nuts and seeds and sweetened with a teaspoon of honey. A small glass (110ml) of pure fruit juice.

Snack: A banana.

Lunch: Low-fat cottage cheese with pineapple, prawns or onion (150g) with a large salad and a crusty wholemeal roll. A bowl of strawberries or a peach.

Snack: A pear and two oatcakes.

Dinner: *Salmon with Honey and Mustard served with new potatoes, green beans and broccoli or a large salad. A baked banana topped with chopped nuts, a drizzle of honey and two tablespoons of low-fat natural fromage frais.

EXERCISE A thirty-minute brisk walk, swim or cycle, plus twenty minutes of strength exercises.

TUESDAY

Breakfast: A serving of no-added-sugar or -salt muesli with skimmed or semi-skimmed milk or low-fat natural yogurt sweetened with a teaspoon of honey and topped with an individual pot of fruit pieces. A small glass (110ml) of pure fruit juice.

Snack: Three cherry tomatoes and a *Wholemeal Scone spread with a little fruit spread.

Lunch: A lean ham and salad wholemeal sandwich or wrap and four cherry tomatoes. A pear and a low-fat natural yogurt sweetened with a teaspoon of honey.

Snack: An apple and a pot of home-made popcorn flavoured with a teaspoon of grated Parmesan.

Dinner: *Chickpea Chilli with brown rice and a large salad. Two *Scotch Pancakes with a small mango puréed and two tablespoons of low-fat natural fromage frais.

EXERCISE Thirty minutes' brisk walking and jogging, or thirty minutes' cycling or swimming.

WEDNESDAY

Breakfast: Two Weetabix topped with four chopped, dried, ready-to-eat, unsulphured apricots and four prunes with skimmed or semi-skimmed milk. A small glass (110ml) of pure fruit juice.

Snack: An apple and small wholemeal currant bun.

Lunch: A 150g pot of low-fat cottage cheese with pineapple, prawns or onion, with a toasted wholemeal pitta bread and salad. A peach or nectarine.

Snack: Two plums and a pot of plain popcorn.

Dinner: *Pork Medallions with Apple and Onion, boiled new potatoes, broccoli and baby carrots or a large salad. A baked apple stuffed with a tablespoon of sultanas and served with two tablespoons of low-fat natural fromage frais and a drizzle of honey.

EXERCISE An aerobic exercise or dance class.

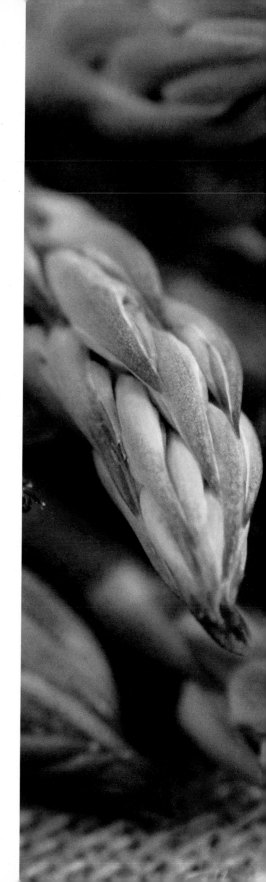

THURSDAY

Breakfast: A serving of porridge made with skimmed or semi-skimmed milk, topped with a chopped banana and a tablespoon of sultanas and sweetened with a teaspoon of honey, if needed. A small glass (110ml) of pure fruit juice.

Snack: An apple and four walnut halves.

Lunch: A wholemeal salmon and salad wrap and a portion of vegetable sticks – carrot, pepper, celery, cucumber. A pear and a low-fat natural yogurt sweetened with a teaspoon of honey.

Snack: An orange or two mandarins, satsumas or clementines, and two oatcakes.

Dinner: *Baked Chicken and Red Pepper Pasta with a green salad. A sliced banana and peach topped with two tablespoons of low-fat natural fromage frais and a tablespoon of chopped seeds.

EXERCISE A thirty-minute brisk walk, cycle or swim, plus twenty minutes of strength exercises.

FRIDAY

Breakfast: A wholemeal English muffin toasted and spread with low-fat olive spread and low-sugar fruit jam. A low-fat natural yogurt topped with a handful of berries and a teaspoon of sunflower seeds. A small glass (110ml) of pure fruit juice.

Snack: A pot of plain popcorn flavoured with a pinch of paprika or a teaspoon of Parmesan.

Lunch: A chicken and salad wholemeal sandwich, with four cherry tomatoes. An orange and a slice of malt loaf.

Snack: A peach or pear.

Dinner: *Mediterranean Prawns and Pasta. A baked apple stuffed with a tablespoon of sultanas and chopped nuts, with two tablespoons of low-fat natural fromage frais.

EXERCISE Thirty minutes' brisk walking, jogging, swimming or cycling.

SATURDAY

Breakfast: A toasted wholemeal English muffin topped with scrambled egg, eight mushrooms, halved and sautéed in a little stock or water, and a grilled tomato. A small glass (110ml) of pure fruit juice.

Snack: Six cherry tomatoes and a pot of plain popcorn.

Lunch: *Egg and New Potato Salad. A pear and a low-fat natural yogurt sweetened with a teaspoon of honey.

Snack: A banana and an oatcake.

Dinner: *Healthy Home-made Fish and Chips, with peas, sweetcorn and grilled tomato. A low-fat natural yogurt topped with a handful of blueberries and a drizzle of honey, if needed.

EXERCISE Forty minutes' swimming or a yoga, martial arts or relaxation class.

SUNDAY

Breakfast: A tin of sardines, sprinkled with a little Worcestershire sauce, grilled on two slices of wholemeal toast, and a grilled tomato. A pear. A small glass (110ml) of skimmed milk or semi-skimmed milk.

Snack: A banana.

Lunch: *Spanish Omelette with a wholemeal crusty roll. A low-fat fruit yogurt.

Snack: A low-fat natural yogurt topped with red berry fruits and sweetened with a little honey, if needed.

Dinner: *Pan-fried Mustardy Pork Chops with mashed potatoes, green beans, courgette and baked tomato. A tropical fruit salad platter – pineapple, kiwi fruit, banana – with two tablespoons of low-fat natural fromage frais.

EXERCISE A thirty-minute brisk walk, cycle or swim, plus twenty minutes of strength exercises.

Week four notes

Day/Time	Food	How do I feel?

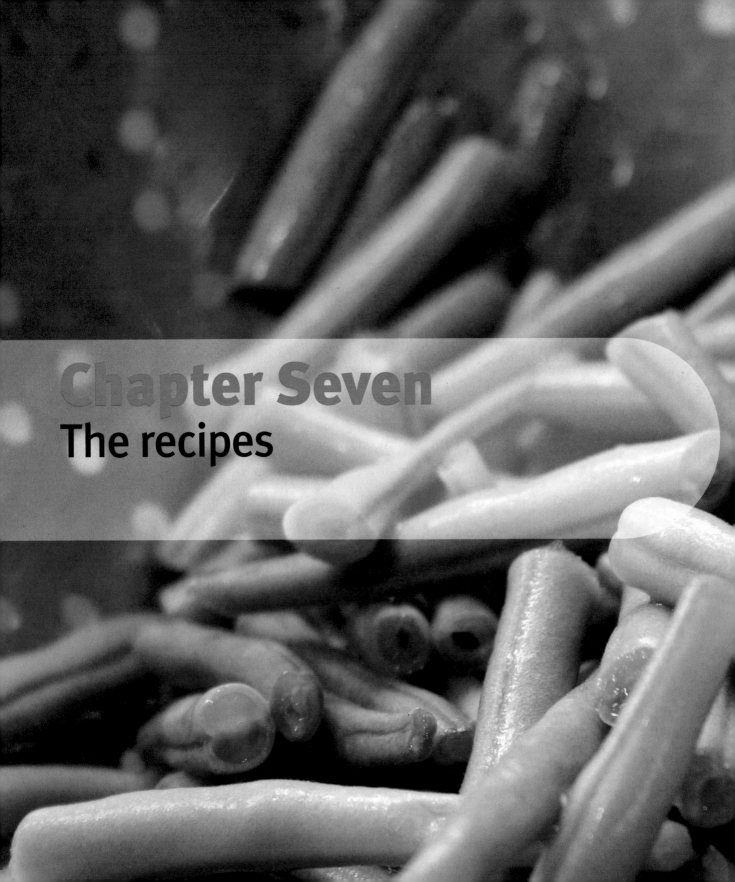

Chapter Seven
The recipes

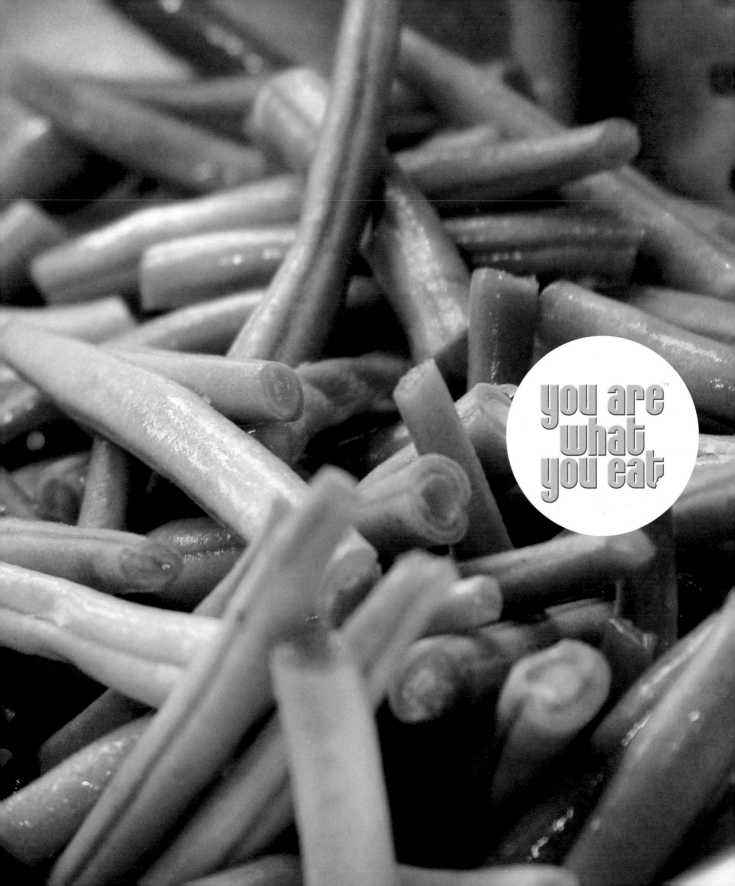

you are
what
you eat

KICK-START PLAN RECIPES

BAKED MANGO CHICKEN WITH APPLE AND ONION RAITA (Serves 2)

1 small mango
1 shallot, peeled and chopped
1tsp mild curry powder or paste
1tbsp water
Low-calorie olive spray
2 small chicken breasts, skin removed
A bag of mixed baby salad leaves

For the raita:

1 eating apple, skin and core removed and finely chopped
1 pinch of chilli powder (or more to taste)
1 small carton low-fat natural yogurt
2 spring onions, finely chopped

1. Preheat the oven to 180C/Gas 4.
2. Place the mango, shallot, curry powder or paste and water in a blender and whiz until smooth.
3. Spray a frying pan with a little low-fat olive spray. Add the chicken breasts and lightly brown on both sides. Transfer the chicken breasts to an ovenproof dish. Spoon the mango mixture over the chicken breasts. Bake in the centre of the oven for 20 to 25 minutes or until the chicken is cooked (the juices should run clear when a knife is inserted into the thickest part of the chicken).
4. To make the raita combine the ingredients in a small bowl.
5. Place a mound of salad leaves and some of the raita on 2 plates. When the chicken is cooked slice each breast into 4 thick wedges and arrange on the salad leaves. Serve with 2 microwaved poppadoms or a portion of wholegrain rice.

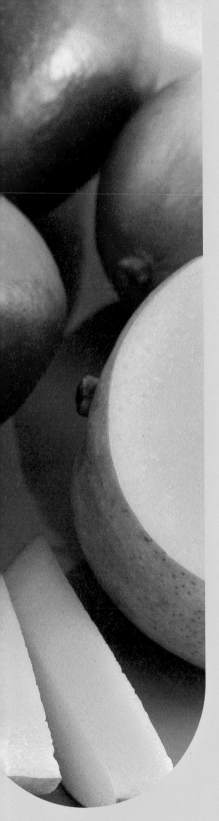

SICILIAN COD (Serves 2)

1tsp olive oil
1 medium onion, finely chopped
1 small can tomatoes
6 stoned black olives, optional
100ml vegetable stock
2x175g thick cod steaks
Handful of basil leaves, roughly torn
Freshly ground black pepper

1. Gently warm the olive oil in a lidded pan and fry the onion until softened but not browned. Add the tomatoes, chopped olives, if using, and vegetable stock and bring to the boil. Add the pepper. Add the fish and spoon the sauce over the fish. Place a lid on the pan and simmer gently for 6 to 8 minutes or until the fish is cooked. The cooking time will depend on the thickness of the fish.
2. Serve the fish on a bed of brown rice with the sauce poured over it, and the basil scattered on top, alongside a large salad or fresh green beans.

VEGETABLE TAGINE (Serves 2)

½tsp olive oil

½ a red onion, finely sliced

¼tsp ground cumin

1 clove garlic, sliced

1tsp chilli paste or harissa paste

1 large carrot, sliced

½ a green or red pepper, de-seeded and sliced

6 ready-to-eat, dried, unsulphured apricots, sliced

1tsp tomato purée

200ml vegetable stock

1 large tomato, cut into wedges

1x300g tin chickpeas, drained and rinsed

1tbsp fresh mint, chopped

Tip: You can reserve a portion of the vegetable tagine and combine with a portion of couscous for a tasty salad for the following day's lunch.

1. Warm the oil in a large saucepan and gently fry the onion until softened. Add the cumin, garlic and chilli or harissa paste and cook for a further minute.

2. Add the carrot, pepper, apricots, tomato purée and stock. Cover the pan and simmer for 15 minutes. Add the tomato wedges and the chickpeas and cook for a further 10 minutes. Just before serving stir in the fresh mint.

3. Serve with couscous (cooked according to the instructions on the packet).

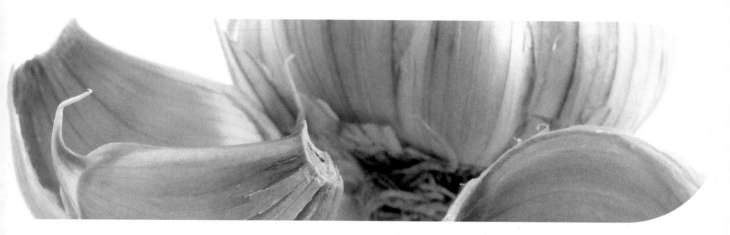

MUSHROOM AND EGG PAN FRY (Serves 1)

½tsp olive oil

100g button mushrooms, wiped and thinly sliced

2 eggs, beaten

1tbsp milk

1tbsp fresh parsley, chopped

Freshly ground black pepper

1 large tomato, skinned, and sliced in rings

25g half-fat Cheddar cheese, grated

1. Lightly oil a small nonstick frying pan and fry the mushrooms gently for a minute. Beat the eggs in a small bowl with the milk and parsley. Season to taste. Add the egg mixture to the mushrooms in the pan and stir over a low heat until the eggs are lightly set.
2. Arrange the tomato slices on top of the egg and sprinkle with the cheese. Place under a hot grill until the cheese is melted and golden.
3. Serve with steamed or boiled new potatoes and sweetcorn.

STIR-FRIED CHICKEN WITH BROCCOLI (Serves 2)

1tsp olive oil

1 large chicken breast, skin removed and cut into thin strips

8 small broccoli florets

½ a red pepper, de-seeded and sliced

4 spring onions

1 clove of garlic, finely chopped

2tbsp water

2tbsp light soy sauce

1tsp honey

1. Heat the oil in a wok or large frying pan. Stir-fry the chicken for 3 to 4 minutes or until it is cooked through. Remove from the pan. Add the vegetables to the pan and fry for 3 minutes, stirring all the time. Add the garlic and the water and cook for a further minute.
2. Add the cooked chicken, soy sauce, water and honey and cook for 1 to 2 minutes until the chicken is just cooked. Serve on a bed of brown rice or wholewheat or buckwheat noodles.

TUNA AND TOMATO PASTA (Serves 2)

100g wholewheat pasta (dry weight)

1 small onion, finely chopped

1tsp olive oil

1 clove garlic, crushed

1 small can chopped tomatoes

1tbsp tomato purée

100g frozen peas

1 large (approx 210g) tin tuna

Freshly ground black pepper

2tbsp half-fat Cheddar cheese, grated

1. Cook the pasta according to the instructions on the packet.
2. Fry the onion in the olive oil for 5 minutes or until softened. Add the garlic and cook for a further minute. Add the chopped tomatoes, tomato purée and peas, and cook for 5 minutes. (If the sauce becomes too thick, add a little water.) Stir in the drained tuna, season with ground black pepper and heat through. Add the cooked and drained pasta and mix together gently. Sprinkle with the cheese.
3. Serve with a large salad.

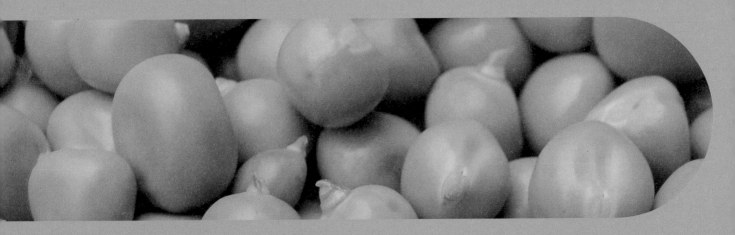

HEARTY BEAN SOUP (Serves 2)

1tsp olive oil
1 medium onion, chopped
1 stick celery
1 medium leek, finely chopped
1 carrot, chopped
1 clove garlic, crushed
1tsp tomato purée
1 small tin chopped tomatoes
½tsp dried mixed herbs
500ml vegetable or chicken stock
1 tin (approx 300g) cannellini or borlotti beans, rinsed and drained
1tbsp fresh parsley, chopped
Freshly ground black pepper

1. Heat the oil in a large saucepan and gently fry the onion, celery, leek, carrot and garlic for 10 minutes until they are softened but not browned. Add the tomato purée, chopped tomatoes, mixed herbs and stock. Simmer for 20 minutes. Add the drained beans and chopped parsley. Heat, then taste and adjust the seasoning if necessary.
2. Serve with warmed crusty wholemeal bread or rolls.

ORIENTAL SALMON (Serves 2)

2x150g salmon steaks
2tbsp soy sauce

1. Marinade the salmon steaks in the soy sauce for at least an hour, or overnight. Grill the salmon until it is just cooked through (about 5 to 7 minutes on each side, depending on the heat of the grill and the thickness of the fish). You could also dry-fry the salmon in a nonstick pan. Take care not to overcook or the salmon will be dry.
2. Serve on a bed of watercress with boiled new potatoes, broccoli and beans.

SPEEDY CHEESY SPAGHETTI (Serves 2)

90g wholewheat spaghetti (dry weight)

½tsp olive oil

1 medium onion, peeled and finely chopped

100g mushrooms, peeled and sliced

1 clove garlic, crushed

1 red pepper, de-seeded and chopped

A small tin of chopped tomatoes

A handful of fresh basil leaves, torn

Freshly ground black pepper

50g feta or mozzarella cheese cut into bite-sized pieces

1. Cook the spaghetti in boiling water in a large saucepan, according to the packet directions.
2. Heat the olive oil in a large frying pan and cook the onions, mushrooms and garlic over a low heat for 5 minutes. Add the red pepper and cook for 2 to 3 minutes more. Add the chopped tomato and cook for 2 minutes. Stir in the cooked spaghetti and the basil leaves. Heat over a low heat for a minute.
3. Season with black pepper, stir in the cheese and serve immediately with a large salad.

GRILLED SALMON WITH SWEET CHILLI SAUCE (Serves 2)

2x150g salmon steaks, skin removed

2tbsp sweet chilli dipping sauce

3tbsp water

2 large handfuls of watercress, or other dark-green salad leaves

1. Using a dry nonstick frying pan, gently pan-fry the salmon until it is cooked, turning once (it will take 4 to 6 minutes for each side depending on the thickness). Add the dipping sauce and the water to the pan with the salmon, and heat.
2. Pile the watercress or salad leaves onto a serving plate. Place the salmon on the top. Pour over the hot sauce so the leaves begin to wilt.
3. Serve with boiled new potatoes, a large halved grilled tomato and broccoli.

You could reserve one of the salmon steaks to serve cold for the next day's lunch.

BAKED CHICKEN WITH HOT MANGO AND PEPPER SALSA (Serves 2)

½ a large mango, skinned and finely chopped
1 small onion, skinned and finely chopped
½ a red pepper, de-seeded and finely chopped
½ a green pepper, de-seeded and finely chopped
Ground black pepper
A pinch of dried chilli powder (optional)
½tsp olive oil
2 small chicken breasts, skins removed

1. Preheat the oven to 180C/Gas 4.
2. Combine the mango, onion, red pepper, green pepper, ground black pepper, chilli powder (if used) and olive oil in a bowl and mix well. Place the chicken breasts in an ovenproof dish and top with the salsa mix. Cover tightly with a piece of foil. Place in the oven and bake for 20 to 25 minutes or until the chicken is cooked through.
3. Serve the chicken breasts and hot salsa with a large green salad and a medium baked jacket potato (maximum size 150g for a woman, 200g for a man).

SCOTCH PANCAKES (Makes 8 to 10 pancakes)

100g wholemeal self-raising flour
1tsp sugar
Pinch of salt
1 egg, beaten
150ml skimmed or semi-skimmed milk

1. Place the flour into a mixing bowl with the sugar and pinch of salt. Make a well in the centre and add the beaten egg. Beat well, gradually incorporating the egg and the milk until you have a smooth batter.
2. Heat a heavy-based nonstick frying pan or flat griddle and wipe with a little oil on a piece of kitchen towel. Drop tablespoons of the pancake mix onto the hot pan, spaced well apart. Cook for 2 minutes until bubbles rise to the surface. Gently turn them over and cook for a further minute.

For a change add a tablespoon of sultanas and a squeeze of lemon juice to your pancake mix, or stir in a tablespoon of fresh blueberries or raspberries.

PORTUGUESE FISH (Serves 2)

1tsp olive oil

2x175g cod or haddock fillets, skin removed

1 small onion, sliced into rings, and separated

1 clove garlic, finely chopped

½ a green pepper, de-seeded and cut into strips

½ a red pepper, de-seeded and cut into strips

1 small can of chopped tomatoes

6 olives, halved (optional)

¼tsp chilli powder (optional)

1 tomato, sliced

Freshly ground black pepper

1. Preheat the oven to 180C/Gas 4.
2. Use a little of the oil to grease an ovenproof dish and lay the fish on the base.
3. Place the remaining oil into a small frying pan and gently fry the onion for 2 to 3 minutes until softened. Add the garlic and sliced pepper and cook for a further minute. Add the chopped tomatoes, olives and chilli, if used. Bring to the boil and remove from the heat.
4. Arrange the tomato slices over the fish, season with freshly ground pepper and pour the sauce over the fish. Cover with foil and bake for 20 to 25 minutes until the fish is cooked.
5. Serve with green beans and broccoli or boiled new potatoes and a large green salad.

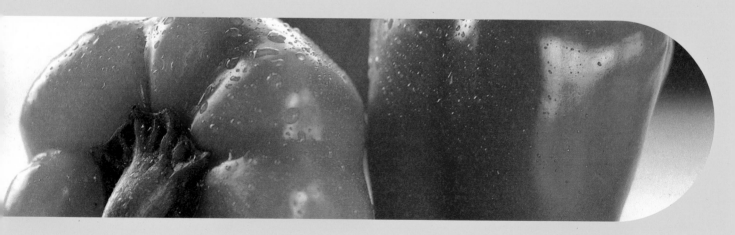

BUTTER BEAN AND VEGETABLE BAKE (Serves 2)

1 medium onion thinly sliced

1 small courgette, chopped

1 red pepper, de-seeded and chopped

6 small mushrooms, quartered

1 large tin chopped tomatoes

1tsp tomato purée

4tbsp water

½tsp paprika, or mild chilli powder

¼tsp cumin

1 tin butter beans (approx 300g), rinsed and drained

For the topping:

1 slice wholemeal bread, crumbed

1tbsp mature Cheddar cheese, grated

1. Preheat the oven to 180C/Gas 4.
2. Place the onion, courgette, pepper, mushrooms, chopped tomato, tomato purée, water and spices into a saucepan and cook gently for 10 minutes. Stir in the drained butter beans.
3. Transfer to an ovenproof dish and top with the breadcrumbs and cheese. Bake in the oven for 15 minutes until piping hot and the cheese has melted.
4. Serve with a large green salad or a serving of green beans and broccoli.

HEALTHY HUMMUS (Makes 4 to 6 servings)

1 large can (400g) of chickpeas

1 small clove garlic, crushed

1tbsp olive oil

1tbsp lemon juice

3tbsp low-fat natural yogurt

Salt and freshly ground black pepper

1. Place all of the ingredients, except the salt and pepper, in a blender and whiz until smooth. Taste and adjust the seasoning by adding pepper and a little salt if needed.
2. Cover and chill in the fridge.
3. Serve in a wrap or pitta bread, with wholegrain crackers, toast fingers or vegetable sticks.

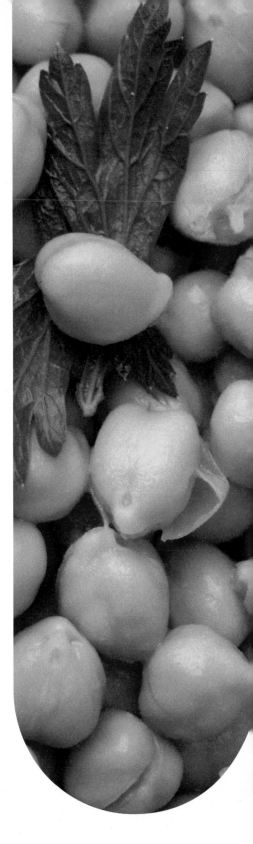

BEAN AND TOMATO HOTPOT (Serves 2)

1tsp olive oil

1 onion, finely sliced

1 carrot, thinly sliced

1 clove garlic

1 large can tomatoes

1tbsp tomato purée

½tsp sugar

50ml vegetable stock or water

2tsp balsamic vinegar

Freshly ground black pepper

1 can (approx 300g) cannellini beans, drained and rinsed

2tbsp low-fat natural yogurt (optional)

1. Heat the olive oil in a pan and gently fry the onion, carrots and garlic until softened. Add the tomatoes, tomato purée, sugar, stock or water, balsamic vinegar and black pepper. Cook gently for 15 minutes. Add the beans and cook for a further 10 minutes.
2. Serve the hotpot topped with a tablespoon of yogurt, with wholewheat pasta and broccoli.

SALMON WITH HONEY AND MUSTARD (Serves 2)

2x175g fresh salmon steaks, skin removed

1tsp runny honey

2tbsp grainy mustard

Ground black pepper

3tbsp water

1. Place the salmon steaks in a nonstick frying pan (no need to add oil). Cook on a gentle heat for 4 minutes, turn over and continue cooking for 3 minutes or until cooked through.
2. Combine the honey, mustard, pepper and water in a small bowl and pour over the salmon. Cook for a further minute. Place a large bed of salad leaves on 2 plates and place a salmon fillet on top. Spoon over the mustard and honey sauce.
3. Serve with boiled new potatoes and broccoli.

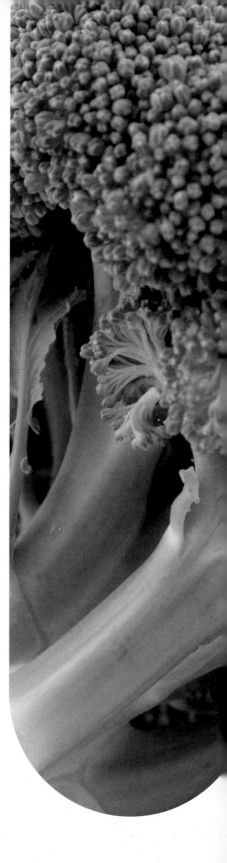

HONEY AND LEMON CHICKEN (Serves 2)

2 small chicken breasts, skin removed
2tbsp lemon juice
1tbsp wholegrain mustard
1tbsp runny honey
8 cherry tomatoes
8 mushrooms, halved

1. Preheat the oven to 200C/Gas 6.
2. Place the chicken breasts in an ovenproof dish. Combine the lemon juice, mustard and honey, and spoon over the chicken. Bake in the oven for 20 to 25 minutes or until the chicken is cooked through. Add the cherry tomatoes and mushrooms to the dish for the last 15 minutes of cooking time.
3. Transfer the chicken to a serving dish with the tomatoes and mushrooms and spoon over any remaining juices in the pan. Serve with boiled new potatoes and broccoli.

SPICY PAN-FRIED FISH (Serves 2)

1 small tin chopped tomatoes
2 spring onions, finely chopped
$\frac{1}{4}$tsp chilli powder
1tbsp flat-leaf parsley, chopped
Ground black pepper
2x175g white-fish fillets (e.g. cod, haddock, hoki), skin removed
$\frac{1}{2}$tsp sugar

1. Put the chopped tomatoes, sugar and spring onions into a large saucepan or lidded frying pan. Add the chilli powder and half of the parsley. Bring to the boil, and season with black pepper.
2. Lay the fish on the top of the tomato mixture and spoon over a little of the mixture. Cover the pan with the lid and gently simmer for 5 to 8 minutes or until it is cooked. The time the fish takes to cook will depend on the thickness of the fillets.
3. Serve the fish and the sauce on a bed of brown rice, with the rest of the parsley sprinkled over and accompanied by green beans and broccoli.

TUNA AND BEAN SALAD (Serves 1)

2 large handfuls of lettuce leaves, torn

1tbsp olive oil

1tbsp vinegar

Freshly ground black pepper

1 small can sweetcorn

2 spring onions, finely chopped

1 small can kidney beans, rinsed and drained

½ a red pepper, de-seeded and chopped

½ a green pepper, de-seeded and chopped

4 tomatoes, halved

1 small can tuna, drained and flaked

If you are planning to take the salad to work you may prefer to take the dressing in a separate container to prevent the lettuce becoming limp.

1. Arrange the lettuce on a plate or in a lidded container if you are taking the salad to work.
2. Combine the olive oil, vinegar and pepper in a small bowl.
3. Put all of the other ingredients, except the tuna and dressing, into a bowl and mix together. Add the flaked tuna. Add the oil and vinegar dressing. Combine gently. Spoon the tuna and bean salad over the lettuce leaves.
4. Serve with a crusty wholemeal roll.

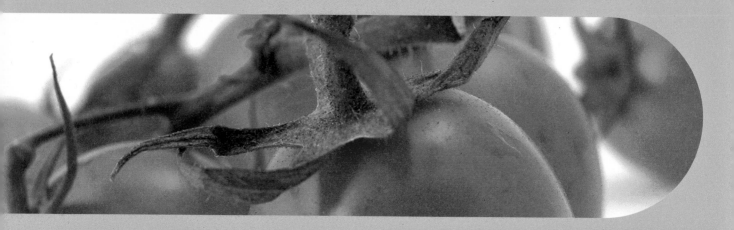

QUICK CAJUN CHICKEN TORTILLAS (Serves 2)

½tsp olive oil

2 small chicken breasts, skinned and thinly sliced

1 medium onion, peeled and thinly sliced

8 mushrooms, thinly sliced

2 tomatoes, each cut into 8 wedges

1 red pepper, de-seeded and cut into thin strips

3tbsp water

½tsp Cajun seasoning

2 wholemeal tortilla wraps

For the dressing:

1tbsp low-fat mayonnaise

1tbsp low-fat natural yogurt

1. Place the oil in a large nonstick frying pan and add the chicken slices. Cook for 4 minutes. Remove from the pan.
2. Fry the onions and mushrooms for 5 minutes until the onion has softened. Add the tomato wedges and pepper strips, the water and the Cajun seasoning. Return the chicken to the pan and cook for 5 to 8 minutes until the chicken is thoroughly cooked and the tomato wedges and pepper have softened.
3. Warm the wholemeal tortilla wraps according to the packet instructions and pile half of the filling onto the middle of each one. Roll up. Place on a plate with a large green salad.
4. Combine the mayonnaise and the yogurt in a small bowl to accompany the tortillas.

If you are cooking for one, reserve half of the filling and a little of the salad and dressing and use to fill a wholemeal wrap for the following day's lunch.

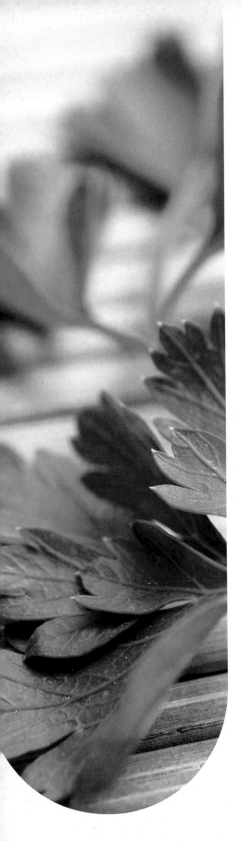

SPICY BAKED BEANS (Serves 2)

½tsp olive oil

1 small onion, finely sliced

1 small red or green chilli, seeds removed and finely sliced (optional)

1 small, red pepper, de-seeded and finely chopped

1 clove garlic, crushed

2 medium tomatoes cut into 8 wedges

½tsp mild curry powder

1 large can reduced-sugar, reduced-salt baked beans

2tbsp water

1tbsp roughly chopped flat-leaf parsley

1. Lightly oil a saucepan and gently fry the onion, chilli if used, and pepper for 5 minutes. Add the garlic, tomato segments and curry powder and cook for a further 5 minutes. Add the baked beans and water and cook gently until the beans are cooked through. Stir in the chopped parsley.
2. Serve on a bed of brown rice or wholewheat pasta.

PASTA WITH FETA CUBES (Serves 2)

½tsp olive oil

4 spring onions chopped

8 pitted black olives, halved

1 small can chopped tomatoes

½tsp sugar

1tbsp tomato purée

1 garlic clove, crushed

4tbsp vegetable stock or water

½tsp crushed dried chillies

2tbsp basil leaves, torn

Freshly ground black pepper

80g wholewheat pasta quills or shells

40g feta cheese, cubed

1. Lightly oil a saucepan and gently fry the spring onions for 5 minutes. Add all of the other ingredients except the pasta and cheese, and bring to the boil. Reduce the heat and simmer gently for 10 minutes.
2. Cook the pasta according to the instructions on the packet.
3. Place the pasta in dishes and pour over the sauce. Sprinkle over the feta cheese cubes.

This salad is also delicious served cold.

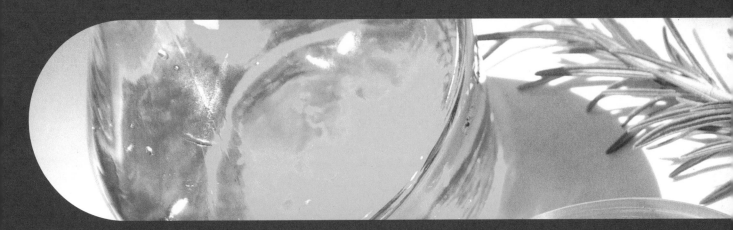

SEAFOOD PIZZA (Serves 2)

1 small tin chopped tomatoes
¼tsp dried mixed herbs or oregano
1 small wholemeal pizza base
2 medium-sized tomatoes
1 small onion, cut into rings
4 mushrooms, sliced
2tbsp sweetcorn
1 can sardines in oil, drained
1tbsp grated mature Cheddar cheese
Freshly ground black pepper
Handful of fresh basil leaves (optional)

If you prefer, you can use tinned mackerel or tuna instead of sardines.

1. Preheat the oven to 200C/Gas 6.
2. Put the tinned tomatoes into a saucepan with the herbs. Boil gently for about 10 minutes until you have a thick sauce. Remove from the heat and allow to cool.
3. Spread the sauce over the pizza base. Arrange the tomatoes, mushrooms and onions over the sauce. Sprinkle over the sweetcorn. Drain the sardines and arrange on the base. Sprinkle over the grated cheese. Season with black pepper. Tear the basil leaves, if used, and sprinkle over the pizza.
4. Bake the pizza in the centre of the oven for 15 – 20 minutes until the base is crisp and the cheese is melted and golden. Serve with a large green salad.

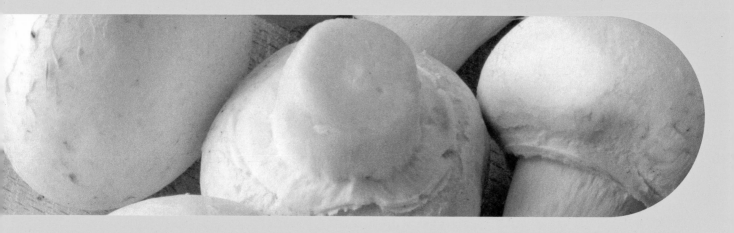

BEAN STEW (Serves 2)

40g pearl barley (cooked for 25 minutes before adding to stew)
1tsp olive oil
1 small onion, thinly sliced
1 garlic clove, chopped
1 stick celery, thinly sliced
1 large carrot, sliced
1 medium parsnip, peeled, core removed and sliced
1 can chopped tomatoes
150ml vegetable stock
½tsp mixed herbs
Freshly ground black pepper
1tbsp roughly chopped flat-leaf parsley
1 tin mixed beans (approx 300g), rinsed and drained

1. Start pre-cooking the barley.
2. Lightly oil a large saucepan and gently fry the onion for 3 minutes. Add the garlic and celery and fry for a further minute. Add the prepared vegetables, chopped tomatoes, pre-cooked pearl barley, stock, herbs and freshly ground pepper and simmer for 20 minutes with the saucepan lid on. Add the mixed beans and simmer for a further 5 minutes.
3. Serve the stew with cabbage, broccoli and boiled new potatoes, or warmed crusty wholemeal bread.

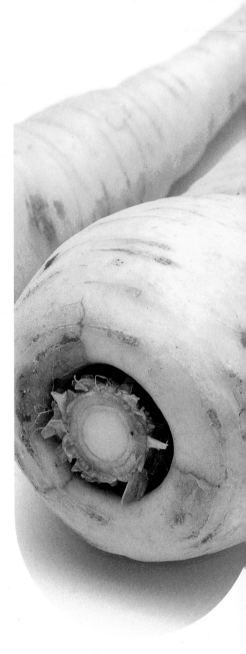

MUSTARD AND ROSEMARY ROAST CHICKEN WITH BABY ROAST POTATOES (Serves 2)

2 chicken breasts, skin removed

2tbsp wholegrain mustard

1tbsp fresh rosemary, stems removed and chopped

1 clove of garlic, crushed

1tsp oil

For the baby roast potatoes:

6 walnut-sized new potatoes, skins left on

1tsp olive oil

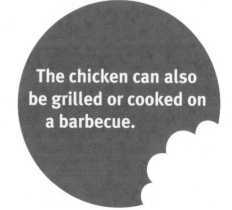

The chicken can also be grilled or cooked on a barbecue.

1. Preheat the oven to 180C/Gas 4.
2. Place the chicken on a nonstick baking tray. Combine the wholegrain mustard, rosemary, garlic and olive oil in a small bowl and spread over the chicken breasts.
3. Boil the potatoes in lightly salted water for 5 minutes. Drain off the water and add 1tsp olive oil to the saucepan. Toss the potatoes to lightly coat in the oil. Transfer to a nonstick baking tray and bake for 40 minutes, shaking occasionally to brown the potatoes. Add the coated chicken to the oven for the last 20 to 25 minutes of cooking time. The chicken is cooked when the juices run clear when pierced with a knife.
4. Serve the chicken with the potatoes and a large green salad or with carrots and broccoli.

CHICKEN STIR-FRY WITH CHINESE LEAVES (Serves 2)

100g instant wholewheat or buckwheat noodles

1tsp olive oil

2 small chicken breasts, skin removed, thinly sliced

2 cloves garlic, crushed

1tsp fresh ginger, grated

1 large red pepper, de-seeded and finely sliced

12 mangetout

6 spring onions, cut into 3cm lengths

125ml vegetable stock

2tbsp light soy sauce

2 heads of pak choi, coarsely chopped

To thicken:

2tsp cornflour mixed to a paste with 2tbsp water

1. Cook the noodles according to the instructions on the packet and set aside.
2. Heat the oil in a wok or large frying pan and stir-fry the chicken until cooked through. Remove the chicken from the pan.
3. Add the garlic, ginger, red pepper, mangetout and onion to the pan and stir-fry for 2 minutes. Add the chicken, soy sauce, vegetable stock and pak choi to the pan and simmer for 2 minutes. Stir in the cornflour paste and heat until the liquid thickens.

Any Chinese greens can be substituted for pak choi.

CHICKPEA CHILLI (Serves 2)

1tsp olive oil
1 medium onion, chopped
2 cloves garlic, crushed
¼tsp chilli powder (or to taste)
150ml vegetable stock
½tsp sugar
1 large (400g) can of chickpeas, rinsed and drained
1 large (400g) can tomatoes
1 medium carrot, finely chopped
1 red pepper, de-seeded and chopped
1 small courgette, roughly sliced
8 mushrooms, quartered
2tbsp low-fat natural yogurt (optional)
Salt and pepper

1. Warm the olive oil in a saucepan and gently fry the onion for 5 to 6 minutes until softened. Add the garlic and chilli powder and cook for a further minute.
2. Add the stock, sugar, chickpeas, canned tomato, chopped carrot, red pepper, courgette and mushrooms. Simmer for 10 minutes or until the vegetables are tender. Add seasoning. Transfer to a serving bowl and spoon the yogurt onto the top, if used.
3. Serve with brown rice and a green salad or fresh boiled vegetables.

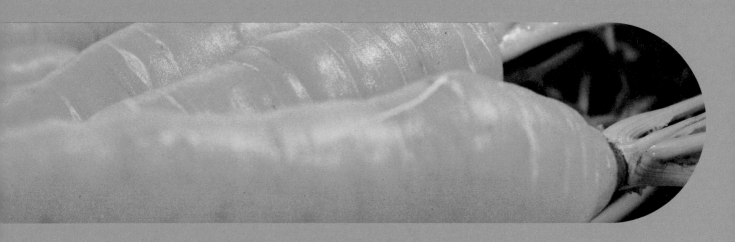

BAKED FISH WITH CHEESY CRUMB TOPPING (Serves 2)

2x150g fillets of fresh or frozen white fish

3 slices wholemeal bread, crumbed

1tbsp Cheddar cheese, grated

1tsp Parmesan cheese, grated

1tbsp parsley, chopped (optional)

1tbsp olive oil

Freshly ground black pepper

1. Preheat the oven to 180C/Gas 4.
2. Place the fish fillets on a nonstick baking tray. Make the bread into crumbs and place in a large bowl. Add all of the other ingredients to the bowl and mix together thoroughly.
3. Press the crumb mixture onto the top of the fillets and bake in the oven for 12 to 15 minutes or until the fish is cooked through (this will depend on the thickness of the fish) and the topping is crisp.
4. Serve with boiled new potatoes, peas, sweetcorn and grilled tomatoes.

CHICKEN AND BEAN CURRY (Serves 2)

1tsp olive oil

1 medium onion, finely sliced

2 small chicken breasts, skin removed and cut into chunks

1 clove garlic, crushed

2tsp medium curry powder, or to taste

150g green beans, trimmed and cut into thirds

5 cherry tomatoes

125ml vegetable stock

1tbsp coriander, chopped (optional)

1. Heat the oil in a large frying pan and gently fry the onion and chicken, until the chicken is browned. Add the garlic and the curry powder and fry for a further minute. Add the remaining ingredients and simmer gently for 15 minutes. Sprinkle over the coriander, if used.
2. Serve with brown basmati rice and a sliced tomato salad.

MEDITERRANEAN PRAWNS AND PASTA (Serves 2)

80g wholewheat pasta (uncooked weight)

1tsp olive oil

½ a small onion, finely chopped

1 red pepper, de-seeded and finely chopped

1 clove garlic, crushed (optional)

¼tsp dried chilli flakes or chilli powder, or to taste

1 small tin chopped tomatoes, drained

6 cherry tomatoes halved

150g cooked frozen prawns, defrosted

1tbsp chopped fresh parsley (optional)

Ground black pepper, to serve

1. Cook the pasta according to the packet instructions.
2. Warm the oil in a nonstick pan and fry the onion, red pepper, garlic and chilli flakes for 2 to 3 minutes. Stir in the chopped tomato and halved cherry tomatoes and cook for another 2 minutes. Add the parsley and the prawns and cook until the prawns are heated through.
3. Drain the pasta and add to the sauce. Serve immediately with a large mixed salad.

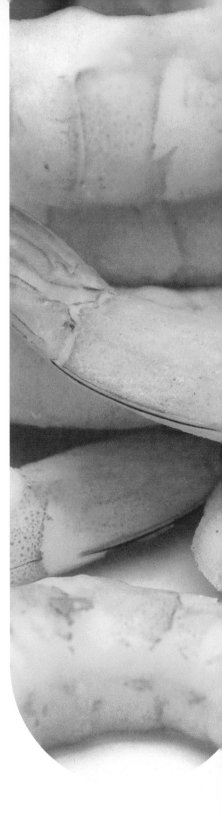

SPANISH OMELETTE (Serves 2)

1tsp olive oil

1 small onion, finely chopped

150g cold cooked potato, diced

2 rashers back bacon, fat removed and chopped

6 cherry tomatoes, halved

4 mushrooms

3 eggs, beaten

Freshly ground black pepper

A pinch of salt

1. Warm the oil in a small nonstick frying pan and fry the onion, potatoes and bacon for about 8 minutes, until the potatoes are beginning to brown. Add the tomato and the mushrooms, and cook for a further 2 to 3 minutes.
2. Break the eggs into a small basin and season with salt and freshly ground black pepper. Add to the pan and cook until the eggs are almost set, then pop under the grill to brown the top. Serve with a hot crusty wholemeal roll and salad.

HOME-MADE HAM, PINEAPPLE AND SWEETCORN PIZZA (Serves 2)

1 small tin chopped tomatoes

½tsp dried mixed herbs or oregano

1 small wholemeal pizza base

2 medium-sized tomatoes

2 slices lean ham

2tbsp sweetcorn

2 pineapple slices (canned in juice), each cut into 8 pieces

2tbsp grated mature Cheddar cheese

Freshly ground black pepper

1. Preheat the oven to 200C/Gas 6.
2. Put the tinned chopped tomato into a saucepan with the herbs. Boil gently for about 10 minutes until you have a thick sauce. Remove from the heat and allow to cool.
3. Spread the sauce over the pizza base. Arrange the tomatoes over the sauce. Sprinkle over the ham, sweetcorn and pineapple. Sprinkle over the grated cheese. Season with black pepper.
4. Bake the pizza in the centre of the oven for 15 to 20 minutes until the base is crisp and the cheese is melted and golden. Serve with a large green salad.

HEALTHY HOME-MADE FISH AND CHIPS (Serves 2)

For the chunky oven chips:

2 large potatoes
Pinch of salt
1tbsp olive oil
Pepper to season

For the fish:

1 egg, beaten
3 slices dried wholemeal bread, crumbed
Pinch of salt
Freshly ground black pepper
300g thick white-fish fillets, skinned
2tsp olive oil

1. Preheat the oven to 200C/Gas 6.
2. To prepare and cook the chunky oven chips: Wash the potatoes, cut into thick chips, leaving the skins on. Boil the potatoes in a saucepan of water with the salt added for 3 minutes then drain and cool immediately under cold water.
3. Place the oil in a large bowl and add the drained chips. Toss to lightly coat them in the oil. Sprinkle with black pepper.
4. Lay the chips on a nonstick baking tray or a piece of nonstick baking paper. Bake for 30 to 35 minutes until they are cooked and golden. Turn a couple of times during cooking so that the chips brown evenly. If they brown too quickly turn the oven heat down a little.
5. To prepare the fish: Beat the egg on a flat plate and put the breadcrumbs, a pinch of salt and ground black pepper on another plate. Dip the fish fillets into the egg and then into the breadcrumbs to coat thoroughly.
6. Place the fish pieces on a nonstick baking tray and spray lightly with a spray olive oil. Bake the fish for 10 minutes. Turn them over, spray again with olive oil spray and cook for another 10 to 15 minutes (depending on the thickness of the fish) until the crumb is golden and fish is cooked through. If they brown too quickly, turn down the oven heat.
7. Serve the fish and chips with peas, sweetcorn and grilled tomatoes.

For a tasty tomato sauce to serve with fish and chips, take a small tin of chopped tomatoes and whiz in a blender or pass through a fine sieve before adding to a small saucepan. Add 1tsp of sugar, 1/2tsp of Worcestershire sauce and some freshly ground black pepper, and cook gently for 10 minutes until the sauce is thick. Transfer into a small serving dish.

SWEET-AND-SOUR CHICKEN STIR-FRY (Serves 2)

1tsp olive oil
1 large chicken breast, skin removed, and thinly sliced
300g bag ready-prepared stir-fry vegetables
½tsp Chinese 5-spice powder

For the sauce:
1tsp sugar
1tbsp soy sauce
1tbsp vinegar
1tbsp cornflour
½tsp fresh ginger, grated
6tbsp water
1 tinned pineapple ring, cut into small pieces
Freshly ground black pepper

1. Put all of the sauce ingredients into a small saucepan and heat gently, stirring constantly, until thickened and smooth.
2. To make the stir-fry, heat the oil in a wok or large frying pan. Add the chicken, and stir-fry over a high heat for 4 to 5 minutes until the chicken is cooked through. Remove from the pan and keep warm.
3. Add the vegetables to the pan with the Chinese 5-spice powder and continue to cook for a further 2 to 3 minutes, so that the vegetables remain crisp. Add the sauce and stir to mix with the chicken and vegetables.
4. Serve with brown rice or wholewheat noodles.

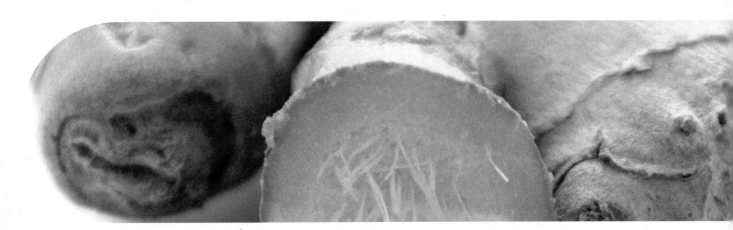

FOREVER PLAN RECIPES

Snacks

If you fancy a change, here are some more healthy snacks you might like to introduce instead of those suggested in the menu plan:

- 100g of cottage cheese, plus carrot, pepper and celery sticks for dipping
- 2tbsp dried fruit and 4 Brazil nuts
- A bowl of fresh fruit salad, with 2tbsp low-fat natural yogurt and a sprinkling of toasted sesame seeds
- A mini currant bun (wholemeal if possible), spread with a little low-fat olive spread or fruit spread if you like
- 2 wholegrain crispbreads such as Ryvita, spread with low-fat cream cheese, plus a piece of fruit
- A banana sliced into a tub of low-fat natural yogurt, drizzled with a teaspoon of runny honey
- A snack salad of some cherry tomatoes, baby cos lettuce leaves, served with 4 olives and 3 breadsticks (wholemeal if possible)

BAKED CHILLI CHICKEN AND FRUITY RICE SALAD (Serves 4)

4 small chicken breasts, skins removed
3tbsp sweet chilli sauce
3tbsp water
A bag of mixed salad leaves

For the fruity rice salad:

1tsp olive oil
1tbsp vinegar
Ground black pepper
1 sachet microwaveable wholegrain rice (or cook 90g from scratch), cooked and allowed to become cold in the fridge
2 pineapple rings (tinned in juice), chopped
3tbsp sultanas
1 small eating apple, washed, cored and finely chopped
2 spring onions, finely chopped
4tbsp cooked frozen peas
A pinch of sugar

1. Preheat the oven to 180C/Gas 4.
2. To make the fruity rice, combine the oil, vinegar and black pepper in a small bowl and mix well. Place all of the other ingredients in a large bowl. Sprinkle over the oil and vinegar dressing and mix together lightly.
3. Place the chicken breasts in an ovenproof dish and cover with foil. Bake for 15 minutes. Combine the sweet chilli sauce and the water in a small bowl. Remove the chicken from the oven. Discard the foil and pour the chilli sauce mixture over the chicken breasts. Return them to the oven and bake for another 10 to 15 minutes or until the chicken is completely cooked through.
4. Place a large mound of salad leaves on 4 plates. Slice each of the chicken breasts into 4 slices and arrange on the leaves. Spoon over any remaining sauce. Place 3 heaped tablespoons of the fruity rice salad alongside.

BAKED PORTUGUESE COD WITH SWEETCORN MASH (Serves 2)

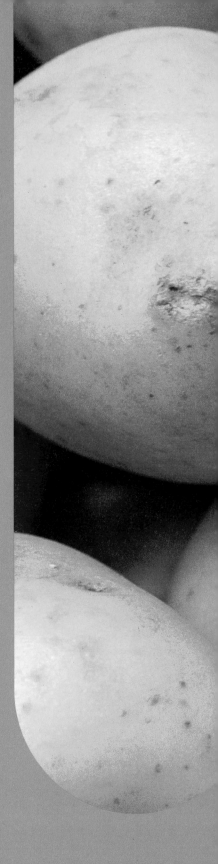

1tsp olive oil

3 medium tomatoes, de-seeded, skinned and chopped

1 small onion, finely chopped

1 clove garlic, crushed

Juice of ½ lemon

2x175g thick fillets or steaks of white fish, skin removed

Freshly ground black pepper

A few sprigs of parsley, chopped

For the sweetcorn mash:

300g potatoes

1tbsp skimmed or semi-skimmed milk

1 small tin of sweetcorn, thoroughly drained

Freshly ground black pepper

1. Preheat the oven to 190C/Gas 5.
2. To make the sweetcorn mash: Boil the potatoes and mash with the milk. Stir in the sweetcorn and black pepper, and transfer to a serving dish. Keep warm if necessary.
3. Heat the oil in a small frying pan and cook the tomatoes, onion and garlic until soft, but not brown. Add the lemon juice.
4. Spoon a little of the mixture into an ovenproof dish and lay the fillets on top. Season them with black pepper and spoon the remaining sauce over the fillets. Cover the dish with a lid or foil and bake for 20 to 25 minutes, or until the fish is cooked.
5. Serve the fish, sprinkled with parsley, on a bed of sweetcorn mash accompanied by green beans.

RAISIN ROCK CAKES (Makes 6 to 8 cakes)

200g wholemeal self-raising flour
1tsp baking powder
½tsp mixed spice
100g olive spread (suitable for baking)
25g soft brown sugar
100g raisins, chopped
Zest of half a lemon
1 medium egg, beaten

1. Preheat the oven to 180C/Gas 4.
2. Lightly oil a baking tray or line with nonstick baking parchment.
3. Into a bowl sift the flour, baking powder and mixed spice. Rub in the olive spread until the dry mixture resembles breadcrumbs. Stir in the sugar, chopped raisins and lemon zest. Add the egg a little at a time until it is just mixed together (you may not need to use all of the egg). The mixture should be rough and slightly crumbly.
4. Place the mixture in rocky lumps onto the prepared baking tray and bake for 15 to 20 minutes until they are lightly golden. Cool on a rack and store in an airtight tin.

GLAZED TUNA STEAKS (Serves 2)

2x150g tuna steaks
1tsp olive oil

For the glaze:
1tbsp wholegrain mustard
1tsp tomato purée
1tbsp orange juice
1tbsp malt vinegar
½tbsp honey
Freshly ground pepper

1. Put all of the ingredients for the glaze into a small nonstick saucepan and simmer until the sauce has a syrupy consistency.
2. Brush the tuna with oil and cook on a preheated griddle or heavy-based frying pan for 2 minutes. Turn the tuna over and brush with a little of the glaze. Cook the tuna for a further 2 to 3 minutes until it is cooked.
3. Place the tuna on serving plates. Reheat the remaining glaze and pour over the fish.
4. Serve with boiled new potatoes in their skins and a large mixed salad.

BAKED FRUIT PARCELS (Serves 2)

2 sliced peaches or nectarines
2 sliced pears
2 slices of pineapple
A handful of raspberries
1tsp honey

1. Place a large square of foil on a baking tray. Place the fruit in the centre of the foil. Drizzle with honey. Fold the foil over to enclose the fruit in a parcel. Bake in the oven for 15 to 20 minutes until the fruit is cooked.
2. Serve each portion with 2tbsp low-fat natural fromage frais.

Tip:
Ring the changes by using other combinations of fruit, and by adding a teaspoon of flaked almonds.

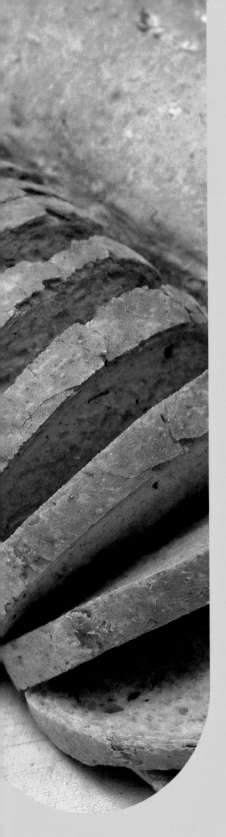

CURRIED LENTIL BAKE (Serves 2)

1 medium onion, thinly sliced
1 clove garlic, finely chopped
1 red pepper, de-seeded and roughly chopped
1tsp mild or medium curry powder
1 tin (approx 400g) Continental or puy lentils, rinsed and drained
1 small can chopped tomatoes
8 French beans, halved
1tbsp sultanas
1tsp tomato purée
8tbsp water
2 handfuls baby spinach leaves

For the topping:
1 slice wholemeal bread, crumbed

1. Preheat the oven to 160/Gas 4.
2. Spray a nonstick pan with a little vegetable oil and gently fry the onions, garlic and red pepper until they begin to soften. Add the curry powder and fry for a further minute. Add the remaining ingredients, except the spinach, and cook gently for 15 minutes. Stir in the spinach and transfer the contents of the pan to an ovenproof dish. Sprinkle over the topping.
3. Bake in the oven for 10 minutes until the topping is crisp.
4. Serve with a large mixed salad and cucumber raita.

CUCUMBER RAITA (Serves 2)

10cm piece of cucumber, skin and seeds removed
1 small carton low-fat natural yogurt
Pinch of turmeric
Pinch of coriander or cumin

1. Chop the cucumber into small dice and add to the yogurt in a mixing bowl. Stir in a pinch of turmeric and the coriander or cumin.
2. Transfer to a serving dish, and refrigerate until needed.

HONEYED LAMB CHOPS (Serves 2)

2 lamb chops, fat removed
Freshly ground black pepper
½tsp olive oil
2tsp honey
1tsp dried mint

1. Rub the chops with the black pepper and the oil and place them on a grill rack. Grill the chops for 4 to 5 minutes. Turn the chops over, and cook for a further 4 to 5 minutes.
2. Combine the honey and the mint and spread over the chops. Cook the chops for another minute on each side. Transfer to a serving dish and spoon any cooking juices over the chops.
3. Serve with mashed potatoes, carrots and green beans and fresh boiled or steamed vegetables.

CRAB AND TOMATO PASTA (Serves 2)

100g wholewheat pasta shapes or spaghetti

1tsp olive oil

Pinch of dried crushed chilli, or a little more to taste

1 small can chopped tomatoes

1tbsp tomato purée

1 small clove garlic, crushed

100ml vegetable stock or water

Freshly ground black pepper

1 large can crab (white meat), drained

1tbsp flat-leaf parsley, chopped

5 cherry tomatoes, halved

1. Cook the pasta according to the instructions on the packet.
2. Place the olive oil in a saucepan and gently cook the chilli for a minute. Stir in the tomatoes, tomato purée, garlic, water or stock and simmer for 10 to 15 minutes until some of the liquid has evaporated. Taste and season with pepper.
3. Just before you are ready to serve, add the drained crab and half of the parsley to the sauce and cook for 1 to 2 minutes until the crab is heated through. Add the drained pasta to the sauce and mix lightly. Transfer to serving bowls and decorate with the halved cherry tomatoes and the remaining parsley.
4. Serve with a large green salad.

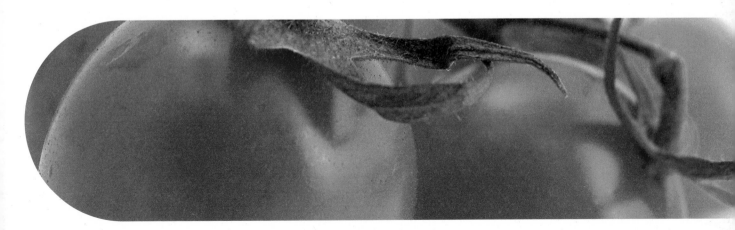

GRILLED FISH AND SPICY LENTILS (Serves 2)

1tsp olive oil

1 small onion, finely chopped

Pinch of ground cumin

¼tsp turmeric

Pinch of chilli flakes, or chilli powder

½ can (400g) Continental or puy lentils, rinsed and drained

2 handfuls of baby spinach leaves

4tbsp low-fat crème fraiche

2x175g fillets of white fish (such as cod, haddock, coley)

1. Heat half of the oil in a nonstick frying pan and fry the onion for 3 minutes until it has softened. Add the cumin, turmeric and chilli flakes and fry for a further minute. Add the lentils, spinach and crème fraiche and cook gently for 3 minutes to wilt the spinach.

2. Brush the fish fillets with the remaining oil and grill under a preheated grill on one side for 3 minutes. Turn over and grill the other side until the fish is cooked. Do not overcook or the fish will dry out.

3. Arrange the lentils and spinach on serving plates and lay the grilled fish on top.

4. Serve with boiled new potatoes, mangetout and grilled tomatoes or a large mixed salad.

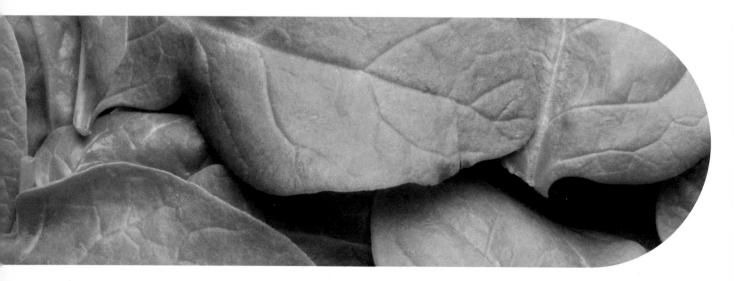

BAKED BEAN CHOWDER (Serves 2)

1tsp olive oil

2 rashers of lean back bacon, all fat removed

1 medium onion, finely chopped

2 medium tomatoes, peeled and chopped

1 medium carrot, diced

1 stick celery, finely chopped

1 small can reduced-sugar, reduced-salt baked beans

Freshly ground black pepper

600ml vegetable stock

1tbsp parsley

1. Place the olive oil in a large saucepan and heat gently. Chop the bacon into small pieces and gently fry with the onion for 5 minutes.
2. Add the tomatoes and carrot and cook for 10 minutes. Add the remaining ingredients and cook for a further 10 minutes.
3. Serve with home-made soda bread (next recipe).

PAN-FRIED MUSTARDY PORK CHOPS (Serves 1)

1 pork chop (all fat removed)

Freshly ground black pepper

1/2tsp olive oil

1tbsp vinegar or orange juice

1tbsp water

1tbsp Dijon or other mild mustard

1. Season the chop with pepper. Brush both sides of the chop with a little olive oil and place in a nonstick frying pan. Fry the chop on both sides until it is cooked. Put the vinegar or orange juice and water in the pan with the mustard. Heat and spoon over the chop in the pan, turning once to coat with the sauce. Place the chop on a serving plate and pour over any pan juices.
2. Serve with boiled new potatoes and fresh vegetables or a salad.

QUICK WHOLEMEAL SODA BREAD (Makes 1 loaf, to be cut into 8 pieces)

500g wholemeal self-raising flour
1tsp bicarbonate of soda
150g pot of low-fat natural yogurt made up to 425ml with skimmed or semi-skimmed milk
1tbsp black treacle
1tsp oats
½tsp salt

1. Preheat the oven to 200C/Gas 6. Lightly flour a nonstick baking tray.
2. Combine the flour, salt and bicarbonate of soda in a large bowl and mix well together. Place the yogurt and milk in a measuring jug and stir in the black treacle.
3. Stir the liquid into the flour and stir together to make a soft dough. Do not over-mix.
4. Turn the dough onto a slightly floured surface and shape the dough into a ball (don't knead it or it will be tough). Transfer to the baking tray. Cut a deep cross into the top of the dough. Sprinkle the bread with the oats and bake in the oven for 30 minutes or until the bread sounds hollow when you tap the base.
5. To serve, cut each of the quarters in half. Soda bread is delicious served with soups and stews. It also freezes well.

STIR-FRIED BEEF WITH BROCCOLI (Serves 2)

1tsp olive oil

150g fillet or sirloin steak, fat removed and thinly sliced into strips

10 small broccoli florets

½ a red pepper, de-seeded and sliced

4 spring onions

1 clove garlic, finely chopped

1tsp fresh ginger, grated

2tbsp water

2tbsp light soy sauce

1tsp honey

1. Heat the oil in a wok or large frying pan. Stir-fry the beef for 2 to 3 minutes or until it is cooked through. Remove from the pan.
2. Add the vegetables to the pan and fry for 3 minutes, stirring all the time. Add the garlic, ginger and water and cook for a further minute.
3. Add the sliced beef, soy sauce and honey and cook for 1 to 2 minutes until the beef is just cooked. Serve on a bed of brown rice or wholewheat noodles.

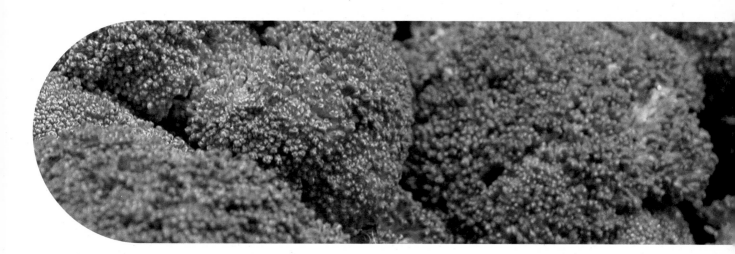

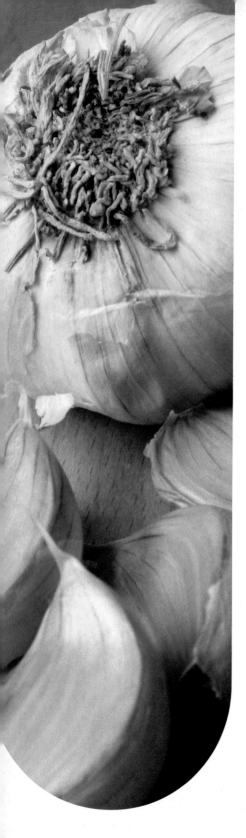

TOMATO TOPPED CHICKEN (Serves 2)

2 small chicken breasts, skin removed
2 plum tomatoes
1 small clove garlic, thinly sliced
Ground black pepper

For the herby potatoes
1tsp olive oil
2 level tsp mild or Dijon mustard
1tbsp chives, snipped
1tbsp parsley, chopped
Freshly ground black pepper
10 walnut-sized waxy potatoes

1. Preheat the oven to 190C/Gas 5.
2. Place the plum tomatoes in boiling water for 30 seconds, remove and peel off the skins. Remove the seeds and slice each tomato into four pieces.
3. Lay the chicken breasts on a piece of baking parchment on a baking tray. Place the sliced garlic on the chicken breasts and top with the slices of tomato. Sprinkle with ground black pepper.
4. Bake the chicken in the oven for 20 to 25 minutes or until the chicken is cooked through.
5. To make the herby potatoes, combine the olive oil, mustard, herbs and black pepper in a small bowl and set aside.
6. Boil the potatoes until just tender. Drain the potatoes, immediately cut each one in half and pour over the dressing. Serve immediately with the chicken and a large green salad.

MUSHROOM AND BROCCOLI PASTA (Serves 2)

100g wholewheat pasta shapes (dry weight)

150g broccoli florets

1tsp olive oil

1 small red onion, finely chopped

1 small clove garlic, crushed

150g mushrooms, sliced

100g low-fat fromage frais

1 level tbsp wholegrain mustard

Freshly ground black pepper

1. Cook the pasta according to the instructions on the packet, adding the broccoli for the last three minutes of cooking time.
2. Heat the oil in a non-stick pan and fry the onions on a low heat for 10 minutes, stirring occasionally. Add the garlic and mushrooms and cook for a further five minutes. Stir in the fromage frais and mustard and heat (do not boil). Add the drained pasta and broccoli and season to taste.
3. Serve immediately with a large salad.

CAULIFLOWER AND BUTTER BEAN CURRY WITH MINT RAITA

(Serves 2)

1 small onion, finely sliced

1 red pepper, de-seeded and chopped

1tsp mild curry powder, or more to taste

12 cauliflower florets

1 clove garlic, crushed

1 small can chopped tomatoes

½tsp sugar

150ml vegetable stock

1 clove garlic, finely chopped

1 small can (approx 150g) butter beans, rinsed and drained

For the raita:

1 small carton natural yogurt

2tsp fresh mint, chopped

Small pinch of chilli powder

1. Lightly oil a saucepan and gently fry the onion and the pepper for 3 minutes. Stir in the curry powder and cook for a further minute. Add the remaining curry ingredients, with the exception of the butter beans. Simmer gently for 10 to 15 minutes then add the drained butter beans and cook for a further 5 minutes.
2. Make the raita by combining the ingredients in a small bowl.
3. Serve on a bed of brown rice accompanied by the raita and a sliced tomato salad.

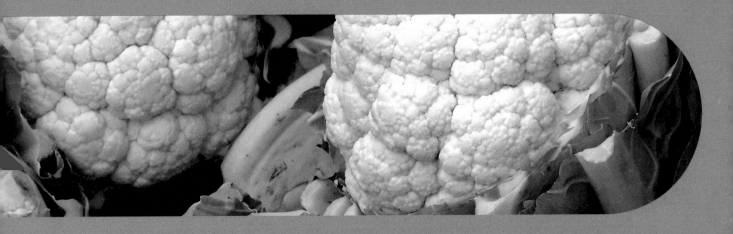

VEGETABLE PASTA (Serves 2)

1 red pepper, de-seeded and chopped

1 red onion, chopped

1 medium courgette, chopped

1 stick celery, chopped

1tsp olive oil

1 clove garlic, crushed

1 small tin tomatoes

1tbsp tomato purée

Freshly ground black pepper

1tbsp chopped basil or parsley

80g wholewheat spaghetti (dry weight)

75g grated mature half-fat Cheddar cheese

1. Finely chop the red pepper, red onion, courgette and celery (or whiz in a food processor briefly).
2. Heat the olive oil in a pan and gently cook the chopped vegetables and crushed garlic until softened but not coloured. Add the chopped tomatoes, tomato purée and ground black pepper and simmer for 15 minutes. Stir in the parsley or basil.
3. Cook the spaghetti according to the instructions on the packet and place in 2 serving bowls. Pour over the sauce and sprinkle with the grated cheese. Serve with a large salad.

This dish is a great way of serving 'disguised' vegetables to children.

GLAZED SALMON WITH WARM ORANGE AND MANGO SALSA

2 small oranges

2tsp soy sauce

2x170g salmon fillets, skin removed

½ a mango, skinned and chopped

¼ a cucumber, rinsed and cubed

1 small red onion, thinly sliced

1tsp fresh mint, chopped

1. Grate the rind from one of the oranges, place the rind in a bowl and add the soy sauce.
2. Cut the skin and pith from both of the oranges and cut out the segments (work over a bowl so that you don't lose any juice). When you have finished segmenting the oranges pour any juice you have collected into the bowl containing the grated rind and soy sauce.
3. Marinate the salmon fillets for 30 minutes in the orange rind, soy sauce and juice.
4. Make the salsa by placing the orange segments, mango, cucumber and red onion and mint into a bowl and mixing together.
5. Heat a dry nonstick frying pan and cook the salmon on each side for 4 to 6 minutes until it is almost cooked through. Add the salsa to the pan and warm.
6. Place a bed of the warmed salsa on serving plates and lay the salmon steaks on top. Serve with new potatoes, green beans and mangetout.

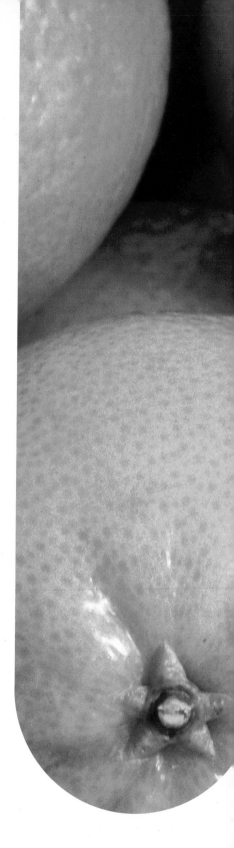

PORK MEDALLIONS WITH APPLE AND ONION (Serves 2)

1tsp olive oil

1 small red onion, finely sliced

1 eating apple, washed, cored and sliced

200g pork fillet, cut into 4 medallions

2tbsp balsamic vinegar

2tbsp water

1tsp chopped parsley

1. Heat the olive oil in a nonstick pan and cook the onion for 2 minutes, add the eating apple and the pork medallions and cook until the pork is cooked through. Add the balsamic vinegar and the water and cook for a further 2 minutes. Transfer to a serving dish and sprinkle with the parsley.
2. Served with boiled new potatoes, broccoli and baby carrots or a large green salad.

EGG AND NEW POTATO SALAD (Serves 2)

2 large handfuls of mixed leaves

A few slices of cucumber

4 cherry tomatoes, halved

5 walnut-sized cooked new potatoes, cooled

1 large hard-boiled egg, quartered

For the dressing:

1tsp olive oil

1tsp lemon juice

1tbsp low-fat natural yogurt

$\frac{1}{2}$tsp sugar

1. Combine the dressing ingredients in a small bowl and set aside.
2. Arrange the salad leaves on plates and top with the cucumber and cherry tomatoes. Cut the new potatoes into thick slices and add to the salad. Arrange the egg on top and drizzle with the dressing.

BAKED CHICKEN AND RED PEPPER PASTA (Serves 2)

80g wholewheat pasta or spaghetti

2 small chicken breasts, skin removed

Ground black pepper

2 small red peppers, de-seeded and chopped

1 onion, roughly chopped

1tsp olive oil

1 clove garlic, crushed

1 small can chopped tomatoes

Freshly ground black pepper

1tbsp chopped parsley

2tbsp low-fat natural yogurt

1. Cook the pasta according to the packet instructions.
2. Preheat the oven to 190C/Gas 5.
3. Place the chicken breasts in the centre of a piece of foil. Season with pepper and make into a parcel. Bake for 20 to 25 minutes or until the chicken is cooked through.
4. Whiz the peppers and onion in a processor until they are finely chopped.
5. Heat the oil in a pan and gently fry the chopped vegetables and garlic until softened. Add the tomatoes and ground black pepper and cook on a low heat for 15 minutes. Stir in the parsley and yoghurt, then stir in the pasta.
6. Serve the chicken with the pasta and a salad.

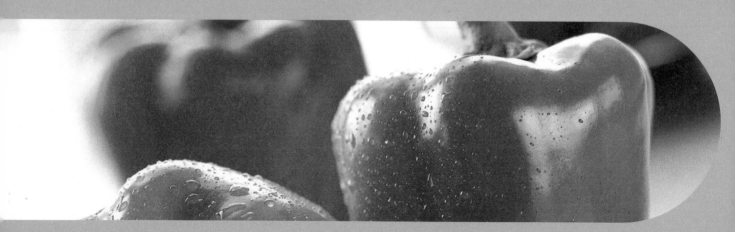

WHOLEMEAL SCONES (makes 8–10)

225g wholemeal self-raising flour (or half-white and half-wholemeal)
Pinch salt
1tsp baking powder
50g olive spread (suitable for baking)
2tsp caster sugar
Milk to mix

1. Preheat the oven to 220C/Gas 7.
2. Sift the flour, salt and baking powder into a bowl. Rub in the spread until the mixture resembles fine breadcrumbs. Stir in the sugar and add sufficient milk to make a soft dough. Turn on to a lightly floured surface and knead lightly (do not over-knead). Roll out to 2 to 2.5cm thick and use a pastry cutter to cut into rounds.
3. Place the scones on a nonstick baking tray and brush the tops with milk. Bake at the top of the oven for 10 to 12 minutes until the scones are well risen and lightly golden. Do not overcook.

Variations:
Apple and cinnamon scones: Add a grated eating apple and $1/2$tsp ground cinnamon.
Fruit scones: Add 50g of mixed dried fruit.
Orange fruit scones: Add the grated rind of a small orange and 50g sultanas.
Cheese scones: Omit the sugar and add a $1/4$ teaspoon dry mustard and 50g of grated half-fat mature Cheddar cheese.
Treacle scones: Omit the sugar and add a tablespoon of black treacle.

Chapter Eight
Food focuses

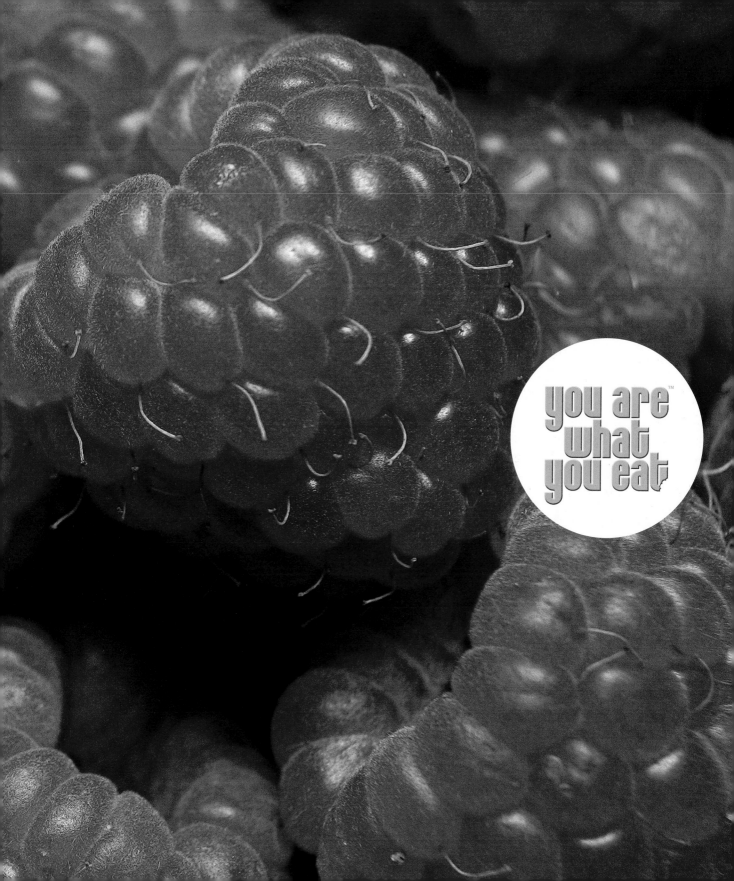

you are™
what
you eat

A healthy balanced diet is the key to all-round health and vitality. Some foods are obviously healthier than others, but nothing is banned (though, admittedly, some foods such as fizzy drinks and sweets have nothing to recommend them, nutritionally!) and balance and moderation are the key.

That said, there are some key foods that, thanks to their amazingly healthy properties, can rightly be considered superfoods.

Just slipping a few superfoods into your diet while continuing to eat junk is not the answer – they're not an 'excuse' for eating a poor diet. But rather than feeling deprived about the foods you know you oughtn't be eating – those saturated and trans fats, salt and added sugars – concentrate instead on upping your intake of these star ingredients:

- Blueberries
- Tomatoes
- Broccoli
- Garlic
- Olive oil
- Salmon
- Tofu
- Tea

Blueberries

These little blue bursts of flavour are one of the richest sources of antioxidants there are. They're packed full of pigments called anthocyanins, which, as well as making blueberries blue, are powerful antioxidants, protecting our body from harmful free-radical molecules.

The antioxidants in blueberries can:

- Reduce damage and 'furring' to your arteries, lessening your risk of heart disease and stroke
- Reduce your risk of cancer
- Reduce the risk of mental deterioration with age, and Alzheimer's
- Delay or prevent the occurrence of age-related eye problems
- Perhaps even slow the general age-related decline in our bodies

Plus, they also contain a useful dose of carotenoids (yet more healthy phyto-chemicals), vitamin C, folic acid and fibre.

An 80g serving of blueberries contains just 59 calories.

You might have heard that phytochemicals in cranberries help to relieve the symptoms of cystitis. Blueberries contain those plant chemicals too, though in slightly lesser amounts.

What to do with them:

- Eat them as a snack.
- Crush them into low-fat natural yogurt or fromage frais for a dessert.
- Add them to fruit salads.
- Sprinkle on top of breakfast cereal, muesli or porridge.
- Add them to apple pies and crumbles for a twist on the traditional apple and blackberry.
- Add them to healthy cakes and bakes.
- Add them to smoothies.

Or try:
Blackberries, blackcurrants, raspberries and cherries – these are also good sources of anthocyanins and other antioxidants.

Tomatoes

Tomatoes' main claim to nutritional fame is their fantastic levels of a plant chemical called lycopene. This compound is a powerful antioxidant, reducing your risk of atherosclerosis, heart disease and stroke, and also of cancer. It's particularly effective at reducing the risk of prostate cancer.

Tomatoes are also a good source of immune-boosting vitamin C. Plus, a medium-sized tomato contains just fifteen calories.

What to do with them:

- Eat them as you would a piece of fruit, cut into wedges – they're delicious sprinkled with a little finely ground black pepper.
- Add to salads.
- Use passata (sieved tomatoes in tins or cartons) to top pizzas, and finish off with slices of fresh tomato.
- Add slices, or tinned tomato, to fish before baking.
- Add slices of fresh tomato to sandwiches, wraps and pitta breads (remove the seeds if they're very watery).
- Cut off the top third of a fresh tomato, scoop out the seeds, fill with a savoury rice filling or break an egg into the hollow, and bake.
- Cut tomatoes into chunks, with some halved small mushrooms and two slices of chopped lean bacon, and cook until the tomato is mushy; serve piled on a toasted wholemeal English muffin.

- Cherry tomatoes are particularly full of flavour, so eat them raw as a snack, add them to salads or pasta sauces, or prick them with a fork (so they don't explode) and bake them.

Getting the best from tomatoes

Most fruit and vegetables lose nutrients when they're cooked, but tomatoes are the exception to the rule. Canned and puréed tomatoes are actually more nutritious than their fresh cousins – cooking them during processing makes it easier for the body to use the beneficial compounds inside them. And adding small amounts of healthy fats (such as olive oil) also makes the lycopene easier for the body to absorb and use. And once again, nutrients have been proven better than supplements – medical studies have found that lycopene eaten in tomato form works better than supplements in lowering 'biomarkers' for diseases such as heart disease and cancer.

Or try:

You can also get lycopene (though not so much) from watermelons and pink grapefruit. They're also good for vitamin C, as are kiwi fruit and blackberries. And all fruit and vegetables are great for fibre.

Broccoli

Broccoli is a powerhouse of nutrients. It's a fantastic source of:

- **Glucosinolates** – phytochemicals that help prevent cancer. The most important glucosinolate in broccoli is called sulphoraphane.
- **Genistein** – a phytochemical that boosts DNA repair, further protecting us from cancer.
- **Betacarotene** – a powerful antioxidant, which the body can also convert to vitamin A, needed for vision, healthy skin and immunity.
- **Zeaxanthin and lutein** – phytochemicals which reduce the risk of age-related eye problems, including cataracts and age-related macular degeneration (AMD).

Or try: Brussels sprouts – they contain virtually the same nutrients and phytochemicals as broccoli. Other green vegetables, such as cabbage, spinach, curly kale and spring greens, are also great for antioxidants, folic acid, zeaxanthin, lutein, iron, calcium, potassium and fibre. For some of these nutrients, they're even better than broccoli, so don't neglect any of your greens!

- **Folic acid** – needed by pregnant women, to reduce the risk of birth defects such as spina bifida in their babies. Plus this member of the B vitamins could also reduce our risk of heart disease.
- **Vitamin C** – supports the immune system, and works as an antioxidant, protecting the body's cells from damage by harmful free-radical molecules.
- **Iron, calcium and potassium** – broccoli contains useful amounts of these minerals, needed to transport oxygen around the body, for healthy bones, and to help maintain a healthy blood pressure.
- **Fibre** – like all vegetables and fruit, broccoli is rich in fibre, which we need to keep our digestive systems healthy. Fibre can also help reduce the risk of bowel cancer.

Tender-stem broccoli is the best source of glucosinolates. Scientists are also trying to develop 'superbroccoli' that's even richer in these compounds.

Plus, an 80g serving of broccoli served 'plain' contains just 30 calories.

What to do with it:

- Buy broccoli as fresh as possible, and don't buy floppy or yellowed sprigs. Or buy it frozen – just bring it to the boil and cook until it's heated through.
- Whether your broccoli is fresh or frozen, don't boil it to death! Boiling means that much of the water-soluble nutrients are lost into the water. And try to do without salt, and let the real flavour show through.
- Steaming is better than boiling. Steam broccoli lightly and eat as a vegetable accompaniment.
- Make into a special side dish by adding a tiny drizzle of olive oil and some toasted sesame seeds (or a squeeze of lemon, or a splash of balsamic vinegar).
- Introduce a novel twist to cauliflower cheese by using half broccoli. Make the cheesy sauce low-fat by using low-fat olive spread, skimmed milk and only a small amount of strong, tasty cheese. You can also make an even lower-fat sauce by using skimmed milk thickened with cornflour mixed with a little milk or water, and flavoured with tasty cheese.
- Add to stir-fries.
- Add tiny sprigs (lightly cooked) to salads.

Garlic

It really is worthwhile learning to love garlic. This powerful little relative of the onion can:

- Lower your level of the harmful LDL form of cholesterol
- Reduce your risk of heart disease and strokes
- Reduce your risk of dangerous blood clots (thromboses)
- Have an antibacterial and antifungal effect
- Research suggests that garlic might reduce your risk of cancer
- Eating garlic regularly could reduce your risk of catching colds

Garlic's amazing health-giving powers are thanks mainly to several useful sulphur compounds, especially one called allicin, which has antioxidant, anti-bacterial and anti-fungal effects.

Getting the best from garlic:

Garlic in its natural state doesn't actually contain allicin – the chemical is produced when the clove is cut or crushed. For maximum flavour and health properties, squeeze garlic through a garlic press rather than chopping it with a knife.

Prolonged heating reduces the effectiveness of garlic, so add it near the end of cooking, or eat it fresh and raw (as in salad dressings).

Buy garlic cloves that are plump and undamaged, and store them in a cool, dark place.

What to do with it:

- Add it to pasta sauces.
- Add crushed garlic to a stir-fry of green vegetables such as broccoli sprigs, curly kale or spinach.
- Roast potatoes and other root vegetables with whole, peeled garlic cloves. The garlic softens and its flavour becomes milder as it cooks.
- Add crushed garlic to salad dressings.

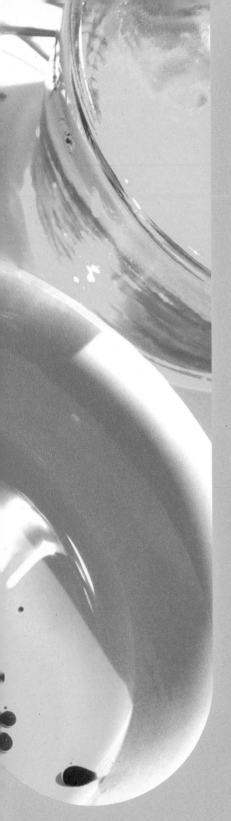

Olive oil

Olive oil is high in monounsaturated fats. These are one of the kinds of healthy fats we all need in moderate amounts. Try to replace as much of the saturated fats in your diet (the kind you find in meat and dairy products) with monounsaturates, and their polyunsaturated cousins.

Olive oil has been found to lower your levels of the 'bad' LDL kind of cholesterol that contributes to clogged arteries. It also raises your levels of the 'good' HDL kind of cholesterol, which ferries fats out of your bloodstream, and helps to keep your arteries clear. All in all, this makes olive oil very good for your heart and blood vessels, and also reduces your risk of strokes. It's believed that olive oil is one of the ingredients that makes the traditional Mediterranean diet so healthy.

The healthiest olive oil is cold-pressed extra-virgin olive oil. This is because it contains higher levels of compounds called phenols, which act as antioxidants. These antioxidants help to mop up the free-radical molecules that damage artery linings, giving olive oil yet another reason to be called 'heart friendly'.

In addition, olive oil is a good source of vitamin E. This fat-soluble vitamin is needed for good immunity, and helps the absorption of other fat-soluble vitamins. Vitamin E also works together with vitamin C to protect our cells from free-radical damage.

Storing and using olive oil

To prevent it from becoming rancid and losing its health-giving properties, olive oil should be stored in a cool, dark place. If you keep it in the fridge it will go cloudy, but the oil will clear once it's returned to room temperature. Olive oil is the healthiest oil for salad dressings, and you can also use it for dipping bread – Mediterranean style – rather than spreading it with butter. Or use olive oil as the fat in sauces, and drizzle a tiny amount on vegetables or baked potatoes. In fact, for most of the occasions when you'd use butter, you could use olive oil instead.

If you fry with olive oil, make sure you don't let it heat to 'smoking point'. If this happens, throw the oil away and start again, as you will have damaged the oil, producing harmful compounds. Overheating also spoils the flavour of olive oil.

Salmon

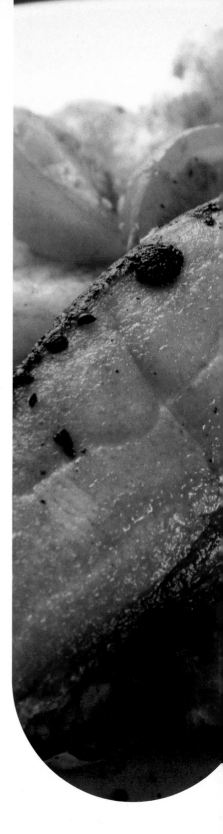

Salmon is a good source of protein, and contains only 2 per cent saturated fat. Oily fish like salmon are higher in total fat than white fish, but most of this is in the healthy unsaturated forms (including those omega-3s that are so good for our hearts and brains). Oily fish are also a useful dietary source of the fat-soluble vitamins A and D.

Eating plenty of oily fish like salmon can:

- Lower your level of blood lipids (fats)
- Reduce your risk of heart disease (including heart attacks) and strokes
- Lessen your risk of Alzheimer's disease
- Slow the rate of mental 'slowdown' associated with ageing
- Benefit babies' brain development when oily fish is eaten by the mother during pregnancy and breast-feeding
- Possibly lessen the risk of depression
- Reduce the symptoms of psoriasis and other inflammatory conditions

Fresh salmon is slightly higher in omega-3s than tinned salmon, but tinned has the added advantage of being rich in calcium, thanks to the bones, which are softened during the canning process, so you can mash them into the fish and eat them.

We're recommended to eat at least two portions of fish a week, at least one of which should be oily (with special guidelines for pregnant women, see page 43), but in reality we only eat an average of one-third of a portion of oily fish a week.

What to do with it:

- Try to choose wild or organic salmon.
- Add flaked grilled salmon to scrambled eggs.
- Add flaked grilled salmon and chopped watercress to an omelette.
- Combine flaked baked salmon with baked Mediterranean vegetables – onion wedges, chopped red pepper, mushrooms and courgette – and a tin of passata for a quick sauce to serve with pasta.
- Make a quick fish pie by combining pieces of baked, grilled or tinned salmon with ready-cooked prawns, with a white sauce (made with skimmed milk and cornflour), a handful of peas or sweetcorn. Top with mashed potato and bake until piping hot.
- Marinate salmon in chilli sauce or soy sauce and grill. Serve with new potatoes and green vegetables.
- Combine wholemeal breadcrumbs with wholegrain mustard as a crusty topping for salmon steaks or fillets. Bake in the oven and serve with new potatoes and vegetables or a salad.
- Bake salmon topped with a parsley or watercress sauce.
- Serve a grilled salmon fillet drizzled with balsamic vinegar with a mixed salad.
- Add cooked flaked salmon to a vegetable stir-fry.
- Combine cooked flaked salmon or tinned salmon with mashed potatoes and finely chopped spring onions to make fish cakes.
- Tinned salmon can also be made into sandwiches and added to salads.

Or try:

Other oily fish such as mackerel, sardines, pilchards, trout and fresh tuna – they are also high in protein and rich in omega-3 fatty acids. Tinned tuna is still good for protein, but the tuna canning process destroys its omega-3s.

You can also buy omega-3 enriched eggs (from chickens fed high-omega-3 feed). Flaxseeds (linseeds) also contain omega-3s, but this is in a form that the body has to convert to the 'active form', a process that is rather inefficient.

Fish-oil supplements are an alternative, and if you are a vegetarian you can also buy omega-3 supplements sourced from micro-algae.

Tofu

Tofu is bean curd, made from soya beans. It's a rather overlooked food, which is a shame, since it's highly nutritious.

Tofu is:

- Low in fat (and the fats it does contain are mainly the healthy omega-3 and omega-6 essential fatty acids)
- Low in calories
- Rich in protein (the highest-quality protein found in a non-animal source)
- Very high in calcium
- A rich source of phytochemicals called isoflavones, which could reduce your risk of cardiovascular disease, and help with female hormone-related symptoms such as those during the menopause

Nutrition scientists first became interested in tofu and other soya products when they noticed that people from countries where a lot of soya is eaten (such as China and Japan) suffer less from certain diseases, such as some cancers, osteoporosis and heart disease. And when the effects of other factors – such as other foods in the diet, and lifestyle in general – were factored out, it appeared that a significant portion of the benefits of the Oriental diet could be down to soya.

Tofu could:

- Lower your level of 'bad' LDL cholesterol, and raise your 'good' HDL cholesterol level, therefore reducing your risk of atherosclerosis (clogged arteries)
- Lessen your risk of heart disease and stroke
- Possibly reduce the hormone-related symptoms of the menopause
- Protect your bones, reducing your risk of osteoporosis

Tofu is a great source of protein for vegetarians, but meat-eaters should give it a try, too. Why not replace one of your meat meals each week with tofu – you'll slash the saturated fat content of your diet.

Kinds of tofu

Tofu comes in two main kinds. Firm tofu comes in blocks (from the chiller cabinet, or vacuum packed so that it doesn't have to be refrigerated) and can be sliced. Silken tofu is softer, rather like cream cheese, and can be used to make nutritious high-protein, high-calcium desserts.

What to do with it:

- Plain tofu can taste bland, so marinate it in a spicy sauce, or a little Worcestershire sauce or soy sauce (reduced salt). You can also buy marinated tofu from the chiller cabinet.
- Stir-fry tofu in a little olive oil (be gentle – it's delicate and prone to break up) and use in Oriental dishes.
- Cut into thin slices, marinate and grill or fry in a little olive oil. Serve as the protein part of your meal. Or serve with toast, grilled tomatoes and sautéed mushrooms.
- Blend or swirl soft silken tofu into fruit purée, and some low-fat natural yogurt if you like, for a nutritious fruit fool.
- Make a tofu scramble from one egg and some crumbled tofu. It will contain less fat and calories, and more calcium, than if you used two eggs. Add some chilli flakes and chopped tomatoes for a spicy twist.

Or try:

- Soya beans – all the health-giving properties of tofu, but with more fibre.
- Soya milk – great if you're allergic or intolerant to dairy, but worth a try for anyone. Look for one that's enriched with calcium, because soya milk is not as rich in this mineral as 'dairy milk'.
- Other soya products – look out for textured vegetable protein (TVP), which can be used as a meat substitute. You can buy it dried, chilled or frozen. Check the ingredients, though, to make sure it's not high in salt or other unwanted additives.

Tea

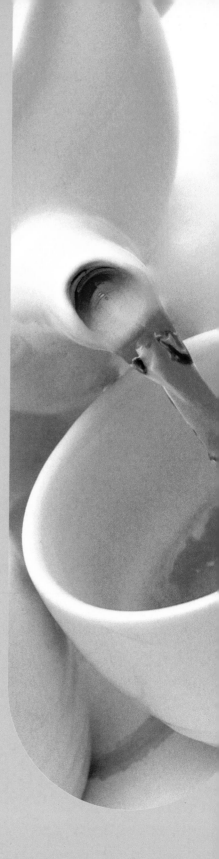

Great news – Britain's traditional favourite drink is good for us! You can't deny the psychological pick-me-up effect of a cup of tea after a hard day's work, but there are chemical reasons for its feel-good factor, too.

The main beneficial compounds in tea are flavonoids, and polyphenol chemicals called catechins.

The phytochemicals in tea can:

- Lower your levels of 'bad' LDL cholesterol, reducing your risk of clogged arteries
- Slightly thin your blood, reducing your risk of dangerous blood clots
- Reduce your blood pressure
- Act as antioxidants, which help to prevent the damage to the linings of the arteries that makes 'furring' and blockages more likely
- Reduce your risk of cancer
- Slow age-related mental decline, and even reduce your risk of Alzheimer's
- Possibly delay other signs of ageing

However, tea also contains caffeine and tannins, which hinder the uptake of nutrients such as calcium and iron from our diet. Because of this, avoid tea late at night if it keeps you awake, and drink it between meals rather than with them, so that you absorb the maximum amount of nutrients from your food.

What kind of tea is best? Although all tea is good, the best effects seem to come from (in order of their polyphenol content) white tea (a special variety, not 'regular' tea taken with milk) and green tea, and traditional tea taken 'black' with no milk. It seems that some of the components of milk bind with the beneficial compounds in the tea, so they don't benefit the body so much.

If you're used to drinking tea with milk, try it black, at least some of the time. Make it weaker, since black tea can taste bitter, particularly if you're not used to it. Try adding a slice of lemon for a different kind of taste.

Or try:

- Rooibos (red bush) tea: Virtually caffeine free, and very high in catechins and polyphenols. It can be drunk black or white, and when taken black tastes less bitter than 'ordinary' tea.
- Herbal and fruit teas: Although these don't contain the particular phytochemicals mentioned above, they are refreshing and hydrating – and a good substitute for sweetened soft drinks. Many are also delicious served chilled.
- Iced tea – ordinary 'infused' tea of any of the kinds we've described, served chilled and perhaps with some ice and slices of orange or lemon. NOT the highly sweetened 'iced tea' you can buy in the shops!

Green and white tea

Research has shown that Japanese people who drank more than two cups of green tea a day had a 50 per cent lower chance of age-related mental decline than those who drank less green tea. It's the high catechin content in the tea that's thought to provide the benefit. White tea (the special variety, not ordinary tea with milk) is even more catechin-rich than green. White tea wasn't tested in the Japanese study, but it would certainly be worth giving it a try.

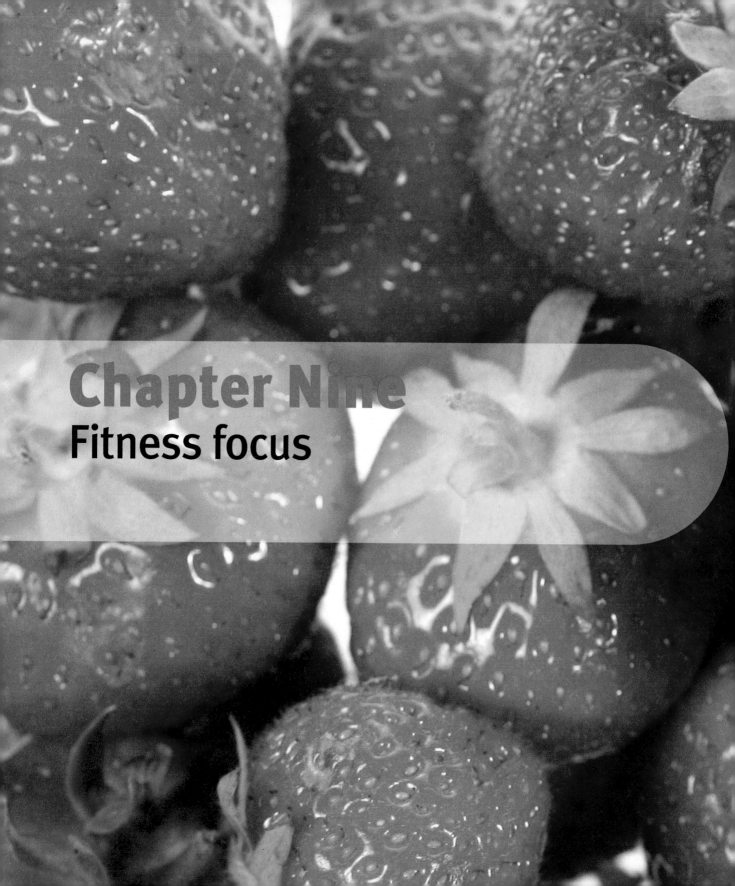

Chapter Nine
Fitness focus

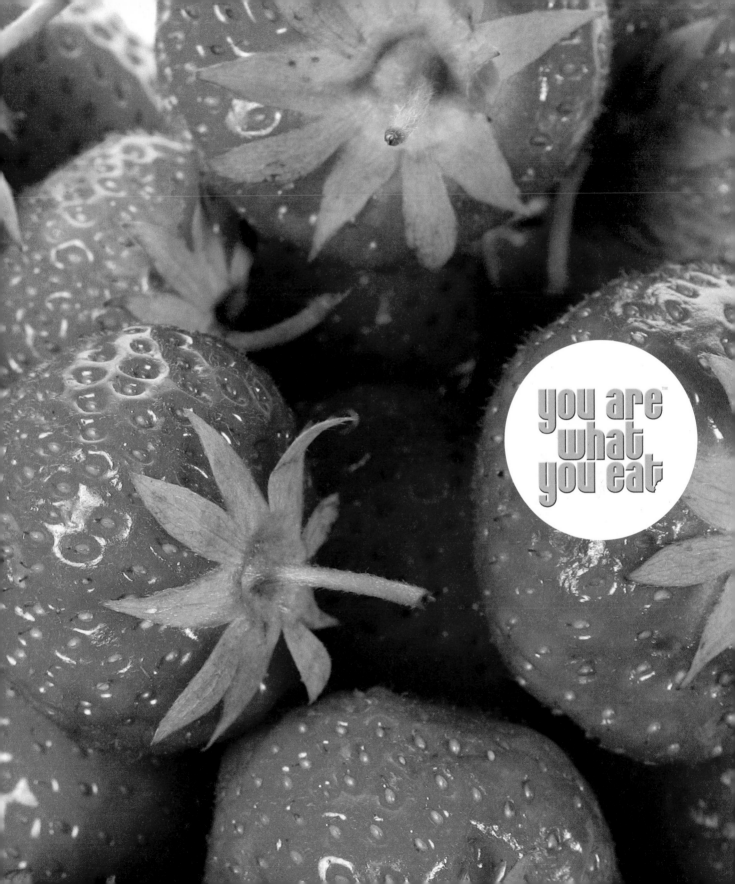

you are™
what
you eat

Fitness doesn't have to mean shelling out on expensive equipment, clothing and gym membership. We've listed just a few 'star moves' that almost anyone can do, for next to nothing.

Star move 1 – Walking

Walking is the exercise we were born to do! It's the most popular form of exercise in the UK, and the best exercise for total fitness novices, as you can start off slowly, then gradually build up the distance and pick up the pace.

What you'll need:
- Some good supportive trainers, or walking shoes or boots for rambling or hill walking
- Suitable clothing if you're walking outdoors

Optional extras:
- A pedometer is useful. By counting your steps, and increasing the number you take over time, you can chart your progress. It's also a great motivator – if you notice your step count is low, you can make an extra effort to catch up by the end of the day.
- A good treadmill if you can afford it, for comfortable all-weather walking.

Once you've got into the swing of things, you need to graduate to 'power walking' – this will turn it into an aerobic exercise, giving your heart and lungs a workout. Swing your arms rhythmically, and stride out! You should feel warm and be slightly out of breath, but still able to carry on a conversation without gasping.

Benefits of walking:
- Good for your cholesterol levels
- Lowers blood pressure
- Boosts bone strength
- Tones the muscles in the legs and buttocks
- Burns calories, helping to lose or maintain weight
- Relieves stress

You know you're really power walking when you're at a speed where you feel it would be easier to break into a run.

Just one mile (1.6km) of power walking can burn up 100 calories. To put that into context, just adding a brisk mile's walking to three days a week could reduce your weight by a pound (0.5kg) in six weeks. That's without any other exercise, and assuming you eat the same amount.

Walking is a weight-bearing exercise, which means it's good for your bones. Provided you wear the right footwear, it's low impact, and kind to your joints.

Choose your shoes

You'll need trainers that are suitable for fitness walking – it's best to ask for advice in a sports shop.

Look for:

- Not too heavy – heavy shoes or trainers can make your calves ache
- Plenty of cushioning under the heel
- Flexible, so that it bends easily when your foot rolls forward
- Breathable, particularly important in hot weather
- A wide base, and support on the inner and outer sides of your ankles, to prevent your foot rolling inward or outward

Walking is easy, but to get the most out of it, and reduce your risk of sore muscles, follow these tips:

- Relax. Don't tense up, particularly your neck and knees.
- Swing your arms to increase your workout. Don't flail them about, but keep them close to your body, and bent at a relaxed 90 degrees, with your hands in loose fists.
- Keep your tummy muscles firm.
- Don't lean forward or stick your neck out as you walk.
- Look forward, not down.
- Don't try to make your strides too long.

Walking is a pretty basic exercise – once you've got the technique right, you don't really need to think about it. To prevent walking from getting boring, just add some variety.

- Vary your route when out walking locally.
- Walk on a treadmill while listening to music or the radio, or watching television.
- Vary the gradient – you can change the setting on many treadmills.
- Try rambling or hill walking – this way you'll get a variety of scenery and gradient, plus the possibility of making new friends if you join a walking club.
- Alternate your walking with jogging. Try walking for five minutes, then a minute's jogging, then back to walking, for the duration of your walk. If that's too much for you, try just picking up the pace a little for one minute in five.

Star move 2 – Swimming

Swimming is one of the best exercises for all-round fitness. It counts as aerobic exercise (benefiting your heart and lungs) and also works all the major muscle groups in the body.

Another plus point is that swimming is extremely easy on the joints, since the water supports your body weight. And although you may feel achy after a particularly long or tough swim, the risks of actual injury are far less than for most other sports.

What you'll need:
- Swimming costume
- Goggles (optional, but useful if the chlorine in the pool stings your eyes)

Start out by simply swimming for as long as you can, giving yourself a break of a minute or so between lengths if you need to. Then gradually try to increase your swimming sessions to around thirty minutes.

Warm up before your swimming session with a walk (could you walk to the pool?) or swimming gently for about five minutes. Cool down afterwards with five minutes of slower strokes.

In order to get the best all-round workout, vary your stroke between front crawl, breaststroke, back crawl and – if you're feeling ambitious – butterfly. If you tend to stick to your favourite stroke, think about taking a few lessons to brush up your technique on the others – and after that, practice makes perfect.

Your body's natural buoyancy provides support in the water, lessening your risk of sport-related injuries, and making swimming an easier exercise if you're overweight, pregnant, have back problems or arthritis. However, swimming doesn't count as weight-bearing exercise. In order to build up your bones, you'll need to find a land-based activity such as walking, jogging, trampolining or weight-training in a gym. Ask your doctor if you're unsure whether these exercises would be suitable for you.

If you're a keen swimmer, three or four thirty- to forty-minute sessions a week will cover the 'aerobic' part of a basic exercise programme. Or you could alternate swimming with other aerobic exercises, such as walking, jogging, running or cycling, if you're worried about getting bored, and to give yourself a weight-bearing workout.

Aquarobics

Another aquatic alternative to swimming is aquarobics. Doing exercises in water provides up to twelve times the resistance of doing the same movements on land, so your muscles get a terrific workout.

See whether your local pool offers classes. Or simply 'run' up and down the pool – you may feel silly, but water running is an excellent aerobic exercise, as well as helping to build and tone your muscles.

Star move 3 – Skipping and Hula-Hooping

We've lumped skipping and Hula-Hooping together, as they're both fantastic aerobic exercises you can enjoy at home with minimal equipment. And although both take a bit of practice, you don't need to take lessons before you can do them.

Skipping

What you'll need:

- A skipping rope (some include a counter). You can pick them up for five to ten pounds. Make sure it's the right length – if you stand on the centre of the rope the point where the handles meet the rope should come to your armpits.
- Good training shoes for high-impact exercise (ask in a sports shop for advice).

Don't be fooled into thinking skipping is for little girls. It's a tough aerobic workout – why do you think boxers rely on it so much? And skipping burns more calories per minute than any other popular exercise except fast running. It's brilliant for your heart and lungs, improves your co-ordination and balance, plus, because it's a weight-bearing exercise, it strengthens your bones, especially in the hips and legs. However, because skipping is 'high impact', you need shoes with plenty of cushioning in the soles.

When you first start out, just skip gently for a few minutes, as though you're jogging on the spot, jumping over the rope every time it swings. You can make your sessions longer as your stamina improves. Allow yourself a rest every few minutes, just walking gently on the spot, so that your muscles stay warm. Start with a ratio of one minute's skipping to three minutes' walking.

Skipping tips:

- Swing the rope using small movements of your wrists – not your whole arm.
- Stay relaxed!
- Keep your back straight and upright – don't hunch over.
- Keep your knees slightly bent at all times.

Once you've mastered basic skipping, vary your workout with:

- Jumping with both feet together. This is speedy and intensive!
- Double bounces – this is skipping with both feet together, but you do a little 'double bounce' for each rotation of the rope. This slows things down, so it's not as tough as jumping with both feet together using a 'single bounce'.
- Figure eights – cross the rope in front of you as it swings, in a figure-eight shape.
- Backwards skipping (both 'jogging' and with both feet together).
- Lifting your knees higher – it gives you a tougher aerobic workout.
- Skipping to music – you can vary the tempo.

Hula-Hooping

This isn't as intense an aerobic exercise as skipping, but it's wonderful for toning the tummy, as it makes you rhythmically tense the muscles all around your middle as you keep that hoop spinning.

What you'll need:

- A Hula Hoop – that's all!

Choosing your hoop

The smaller the hoop, the trickier it is to keep in the air, as it will spin faster. As a rough guideline, rest the rim of the hoop on the floor in front of you – it should come up to about 10cm (4 inches) above your waist. If you're a beginner, you might find a bigger hoop easier, and if you want to make things more challenging, try a smaller one. You can also buy weighted hoops, which make you work a little harder.

Getting started

Start by stepping into the hoop, and holding it just above waist level. Then start it spinning, and keep it spinning by moving your hips backwards and forwards (don't try to move them in a circle to make the hoop do the same – this just makes things harder!).

Then you can vary your routine:

- Stand with one foot slightly forward (this makes it easier)
- Stand with both feet together (this makes it harder)
- Vary your arm position – hold them out to the sides, straight above your head, wave them around to intensify the effort you put in
- Speed up and slow down

Star move 4 – Press-ups and crunches

Press-ups and crunches are varieties of resistance (strength) training. They'll improve your upper-body strength (press-ups) and tone your stomach (crunches). All forms of strength training increase your proportion of muscle mass to fat mass, boosting your metabolic rate so that you'll burn more calories even when you're not exercising.

And for both of these exercises, you need no equipment whatsoever.

Press-ups

Everyone knows how to do press-ups (or push-ups), but many people don't do them properly, so they don't gain the full benefits.

There are two versions. For the tough version – full press-ups – you rest your hands and your toes on the floor, with your legs stretched out straight. For much easier 'half press-ups', you rest on your hands and knees, with your feet crossed at the ankles and raised behind you.

Start in the 'down' position, with your palms on the floor, slightly to the side and in front of your shoulders. Then slowly straighten your arms and raise your body until you are resting on your hands and your toes or knees. Then bend your elbows and lower your body so that your chest almost touches the ground, before slowly straightening your arms again.

Press-up tips:

- Don't lock your elbows when you straighten your arms
- Don't let your chest touch the floor between press-ups
- Keep your tummy tucked in (but not totally tensed); this means that you work your core muscles, not just your arms
- Breathe out as you come up, and in as you go down

Crunches

Crunches are the exercise most commonly performed badly! But if you do them correctly, they're great for strong core muscles and tummy-toning. Strong abdominal muscles (abs) also make you less likely to suffer from a bad back.

Start off by lying on your back, with your feet hip-width apart, your knees bent and your feet flat on the floor. Rest your fingertips lightly on your ears, with your elbows out to the sides, pointing slightly forwards. Then gently curl up – pause – then return to the ground. Each 'up and down' should take about four or five seconds.

Crunch tips:

- Keep the movements slow and controlled
- Breathe out as you come up, and in as you go down
- Concentrate on 'shortening' your stomach, not curling your back
- Don't yank your body up by your ears!
- Keep your neck in line with your back, and keep a gap between your chin and your chest – imagine you are trying to hold a tennis ball under your chin

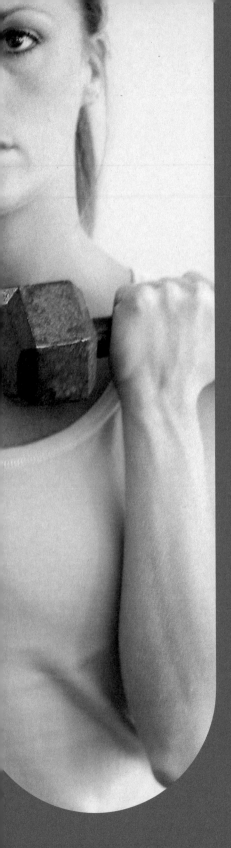

Star move 5 – Hand and ankle weights

You can replicate many of the exercises you perform at the gym in your own home, using hand and ankle weights. While a machine at the gym can generally only be used for one or two exercises, 'free weights' are much more versatile and can be used for a whole variety of moves, and you don't even have to leave your own home.

Hand weights are basically little dumbbells. Ankle weights are fitted around your ankles, usually using Velcro and adjustable straps. They are generally padded to make them more comfortable, and the smaller, lighter ankle weights can also be used as wrist weights.

What you'll need:
- A pair of hand weights (or you could improvise using tin cans or bottles of water)
- A pair of ankle weights

You can pick up a pair of basic hand weights for under ten pounds, and ankle weights for even less. You can also buy sets of hand weights, ranging from really light to heftier weights. This is really useful – some of the muscles in your arms and shoulders are naturally stronger than others, and so you need to work them with heavier weights than the weaker muscles. Also, if you buy a set of weights, you can move up to your bigger weights as your muscles grow stronger.

Some simple weights exercises

Biceps curls

This is probably the most familiar hand-weights exercise, and you'll soon see and feel benefits if you do it regularly, and use the proper technique.

How to: Hold your hand weights in front of your thighs, with your arms almost straight (don't lock your elbows). Bend your elbows so that you lift the weights up and your knuckles touch your shoulders. Slowly lower the weights to the starting position. That's one repetition of the exercise.

Triceps extensions

While biceps curls work the large muscles at the front of your upper arms (your biceps), this exercise works the smaller muscles (triceps) at the back of your upper arms. The triceps are smaller than the biceps, so you'll find it easier to use lighter weights for this exercise. Unlike the biceps curl, you work one arm, then swap over to exercise the other one.

How to: It takes a moment or two to get into the starting position. Hold a hand weight in one hand. Bend the arm, so that the hand and the weight are by your shoulders (as at the top of the biceps curl move). Now cup the elbow of the hand holding the weight with your other hand – this hand is going to support the arm that's doing the work.

Now lift the arm with the weight so that your elbow points towards the ceiling and your shoulder drops down – the weight should now be behind your ear. You're now in the starting position! Extend and straighten the lifting arm up towards the ceiling. Then slowly bend the arm back to the starting position – that's one repetition of the exercise. There's a great temptation to arch your back as you do this exercise – make sure you resist it.

Side lifts (1)

This exercise works your outer thigh muscles.

How to: Put on your ankle weights. Lie down on your side, leaning on your elbow, with your head resting on your hand. Your body and legs should be in a straight line, with one leg on top of the other. Slowly raise the top leg, then lower it. (You may find it easier if you bend your lower leg slightly, to give you more stability.) This is one repetition of the exercise.

When you've worked one leg, roll over and repeat for the other side.

Side lifts (2)

This exercise works your inner thigh muscles.

How to: Put on your ankle weights. Lie down on your side, leaning on your elbow, with your head resting on your hand. Your bottom leg should be extended in a straight line, and the other leg should be bent, with the foot placed behind the knee of the bottom leg.

Now slowly lift the bottom (straight) leg a few inches, and lower it again. This is one repetition of the exercise. When you've worked one leg, roll over and repeat for the other side.

Weights tips:

- You should just be able to do ten repetitions of the exercise you are attempting, without a rest.
- Don't try to lift weights that are too heavy. If your weights are too heavy, your technique will suffer, and you are more likely to injure yourself.
- If you find the exercises working your legs too tough, take off your ankle weights. Training shoes can be quite heavy, and can provide enough weight for a beginner. Once your legs are stronger, you'll be able to use the ankle weights.
- Your moves should be slow and controlled.
- Don't swing your weights – this reduces the benefit and you could also pull a muscle.
- Don't lock your elbows as you straighten your arms.
- Don't lock your knees as you straighten your legs.
- Even though you're working your arms or legs, keep your stomach muscles firm as well.
- If, as you get stronger, you find that your hand weights aren't heavy enough any more, put your ankle weights around your wrists as well.

We've given you only a tiny selection of exercises using hand and ankleweights, working only a few of your upper- and lower-body muscles, to whet your appetite and get you started. You can also use hand and ankle weights to work your shoulders, back, buttocks and ankles – ask for advice at a gym or buy or borrow a good exercise manual if you want to learn more.

APPENDIX

EXAMPLE FOOD DIARY

Date and time	Food	Comments
Monday 1 February		
7.30	Bowl of cornflakes with semi-skimmed milk and 2tsp sugar	My usual work-day breakfast.
	Slice of white toast, spread with sunflower margarine and marmalade	
	Cup of coffee (white with 1tsp sugar)	
10.30	Cup of coffee (white, 1 sugar)	
	Danish pastry	Felt hungry, so bought this from the 'sandwich girl' who visits our office. Felt guilty after I ate it.
12.30	Cheese and pickle sandwich, on white bread	Lunch bought from the sandwich girl.
	Low-fat strawberry-flavour yogurt	
	Packet of crisps	
	Can of diet lemonade	Felt tired afterwards.
3.45	Cup of coffee (white, 1 sugar)	
	3 chocolate biscuits	Wasn't really hungry, just felt 'munchy'.

6.30	2-finger chocolate wafer biscuit	Wouldn't normally raid the biscuit barrel at this time, but fancied something to keep me going, because I'd be eating later tonight.
7.45	Large glass of white wine	Waiting at the pizza restaurant for everyone to arrive for our girly night out.
8.00	2 pieces garlic bread	I know it's not healthy, but I love it!
	½ cheese and pepperoni pizza	
	Small salad bowl (including coleslaw and potato salad)	Didn't really need this, but it came as part of a 'meal deal'.
	3 large glasses white wine	
	Slice of treacle tart with cream	Everyone had a dessert, and I couldn't resist, even though I don't have 'pudding' at home.
	2 cups coffee (white, 1 sugar)	Felt full and bloated.
		Later in the evening I felt 'tired but wired'. I think I may regret this tomorrow.

This is just an example of someone's food diary before they started out on our Kick-start Plan. Let's call her Lucy . . .

Food diary analysis

Breakfast:

Cereal and toast is the 'usual breakfast' for a lot of us, but a bowl of porridge made with semi-skimmed milk, topped with some chopped nuts, would have sustained Lucy for longer, so she wouldn't have been so hungry mid-morning and succumbed to the temptation of the sticky pastry. Also, wholemeal toast would have boosted her fibre intake, and a spread that's high in monounsaturates (such as an olive spread) is healthier than sunflower spread. A little marmalade is allowable in the plan, but Lucy will need to make sure it's a low-sugar high-fruit variety. She should also try to wean herself off sugar in her coffee, as her sugar intake is rather high. In fact, she might feel better if she cuts down her coffee intake, too. A small glass of orange juice instead would have boosted her vitamin C intake, and counted as one portion towards her 'five-a-day'.

Morning snack:

If she'd had a more filling and higher-fibre breakfast, Lucy probably wouldn't have had the Danish pastry – or the guilt that came with it. A piece of fruit such as an apple would have boosted her fibre and vitamin account, added to her 'five-a-day' count, and soothed any 'snackish' feelings she may get if she's used to having something to eat at Elevenses.

Lunch:

Lucy's sandwich is low in fibre and high in saturated fat (thanks to the cheese). A better choice would have been a sandwich using wholemeal bread, with a low-fat protein filling such as chicken or turkey, and plenty of salad. Although the yogurt was low-fat, bought yogurts contain a lot of sugar. A tub of low-fat natural yogurt, with some fresh berries, would have been healthier. The packet of crisps is obviously high in salt and fat. And although it's low-calorie, the fizzy drink is nothing but fizzy sweetened water, and contributes nothing to Lucy's nutrient intake. If she brought her lunch from home, Lucy could have eaten much more healthily.

Afternoon snack:

Lucy ate through habit rather than hunger. She could have been prepared for the mid-afternoon munchies, and brought a healthy handful of unsalted nuts and raisins to fill that gap.

Early evening snack:

It's understandable that Lucy would feel hungry now, particularly since she's eating later than usual, and her sugary snack earlier in the afternoon would have only sustained her for a short time. She would have been better having a slow-release snack, such as a couple of oatcakes spread with low-fat soft cheese, providing complex starchy carbohydrates with a little protein.

At the restaurant:

Sometimes it's not a wise idea to drink alcohol before a meal, as it can weaken your self-control, so you forget all your good intentions.

This kind of meal (indeed, a lot of the things Lucy ate) wouldn't be seen in our Kick-start Plan. But in the maintenance phase she'd be allowed the occasional 'lapse' from totally healthy eating, such as for this girly night out. She should just make healthier choices.

Garlic bread is made from white bread (not wholemeal), and it oozes butter, so it's high in saturated fat. Bearing this in mind, Lucy could perhaps have had just one piece of garlic bread (this is a treat, after all), and given the rest of her portion to her friends. She could have had the thin-crust pizza, and asked for maximum vegetables (no meat toppings) and only the tiniest sprinkling of cheese.

She should have had as big a salad as she could, but held on the coleslaw and potato salad, to minimise her fat intake. And for dessert, she should have chosen sorbet or ice cream. Or, if she couldn't resist something sticky and decadent, she could have asked for two spoons and shared it with a friend.

Lucy drank quite a lot more alcohol than the recommended maximum for a woman, and should have stuck to no more than 3 units (see page 72). Even if she didn't drink during the rest of the week, it's not healthy to save up your weekly allowance – this counts as binge drinking.

Looking back over the day, we can see that Lucy is drinking quite a lot of coffee, and felt 'wired but tired' at the end of the day, just after her two coffees at the restaurant. The 'tired' feeling wasn't helped by the heavy meal and all that wine. And she'd probably feel less wired and jittery if she swapped at least some of those coffees for non-caffeinated drinks.

YOUR FOOD DIARY

Copy into a notebook, or photocopy as many times as you like.

Date and time	Food	Comments

INDEX